ABOUT THE AUTHORS

Dr Danny Penman is an award-winning investigative journalist. He currently writes features for the *Daily Mail*, having previously worked for the *BBC*, *New Scientist* and the *Independent* newspaper. He is co-author of the bestselling *Mindfulness: A practical guide to finding peace in a frantic world*, and has been a keen meditator for over 30 years. **Vidyamala Burch** is the founder of Breathworks, an internationally respected mindfulness organisation with trainers in 15 countries. She is author of *Living Well with Pain and Illness: Using mindfulness to free yourself from suffering.* Breathworks grew out of Vidyamala's personal experience of using mindfulness and meditation to manage her own chronic pain.

ADVANCE PRAISE FOR *MINDFULNESS FOR HEALTH*

'This book provides an extremely effective and elegant mind–body approach to healing for people dealing with the potentially hugely eroding effects of chronic pain and illness in their lives. The Breathworks approach to Mindfulness-Based Pain Management (MBPM) is the most comprehensive, in-depth, scientifically up-to-date and user-friendly approach to learning the *how* of living with chronic pain and reclaiming one's life that I know of. This is not surprising, given the authors' direct personal experience with severe injury, extensive rehabilitation, and discovering the need to take charge of their own recovery to optimize long-term wellbeing. Highly recommended'

Jon Kabat-Zinn, PhD
author of *Full Catastrophe Living* and *Coming to Our Senses*
Professor Emeritus of the University of Massachusetts Medical School

'Written by authors for whom pain is no stranger, and with many years' experience of mindfulness, this wonderful book carries readers through ways of engaging with pain. All the mindfulness practices are described with gentleness and compassion, helping sufferers shift from anger and fighting with pain, to becoming accepting and compassionate to pain. In a world of much suffering, this book is a gift of wisdom and practical help'

Professor Paul Gilbert, PhD, OBE
author of *The Compassionate Mind* and *Mindful Compassion*
Derbyshire Healthcare NHS Foundation Trust, UK

'If you have chronic pain or another persistent health problem, if you struggle, feel stuck or feel alone, read and follow this book. It will encourage, guide and liberate you. This generously conceived and practically organised book will help you, just as it says, to find your new chances, watch your suffering dissolve, find pleasure in small things, and to learn that you are not alone'

Lance M. McCracken, PhD
Professor of Behavioural Medicine,
King's College London
Psychology Lead, INPUT Pain Management Service,
Guy's and St Thomas' NHS Foundation Trust, London

'This book will be an excellent resource for people in the community who live with pain and long-term health conditions, and also for those health-care professionals who support them.

Persistent pain is one of the most challenging health conditions to understand, treat and to manage. What I like most about *Mindfulness for Health* is that it's been written by authors who actually live with pain, and it provides simple, easy-to-understand, practical ways to manage it. I know many readers will benefit from using it as a 'buddy' whilst on their journey living with pain'

Peter Moore
co-author of the *Pain Toolkit*
www.paintoolkit.org

'The authors manage to tackle one of the most fundamental of human problems, suffering with pain, in a practical, lucid and kind manner. They draw on their own experience, and on accounts of others' struggles and discoveries, in exploring mindfulness, as well as on Buddhism and findings from medicine and neuroscience. Their descriptions use effortlessly integrated language of mind and body, with neither the bossiness of some self-help texts nor the mystification and fake positivity of others. Through simple exercises, well explained and prepared, and with a parallel CD, they guide the reader through the principles and practice of mindfulness applied to pain, and towards self-understanding, gentle control and connectedness'

Dr Amanda C de C Williams
Reader in Clinical Health Psychology
University College London

'Being challenged by ongoing illness or pain is not for the faint-hearted. And neither is mindfulness; it takes some courage, time and commitment to practise. However, mindfulness does offer us a way of rediscovering our capacity for ease, choice and participation in life, no matter what our circumstances.

Vidyamala and Danny have written an inspiring book which can be a vital guide on your journey to integrating mindfulness into your life. It is alive with heart-warming stories and practical and engaging ways of managing your distress and finding more joy, peace, wisdom and compassion for yourself and others – from day one of this excellent programme. It is a guidebook for thriving and not just surviving each day'

Timothea Goddard
MBSR teacher, Psychotherapist – Openground, Australia

'This book is an excellent resource for starting a journey with mindfulness approaches to pain and health problems. It draws on the authors' own knowledge and experience of pain and ill health, so builds confidence in the reader's mind that the authors know and understand the journey only too well, and the changes needed to lessen suffering. The carefully guided weekly instructions that form the eight-week course make mindfulness practice feasible even for those not completely committed or enthusiastic. The numerous examples of people using the course for their illness, stress or pain guide the individual as they progress and provide encouragement to stay with the practice to sustain change.

The evidence drawn from numerous scientific sources helps support the book's content and is invaluable for 'disbelievers'. This book will be enormously valuable for numerous clinicians and practitioners in helping them develop mindfulness, and frame and deliver mindfulness programmes for patients with long-term health problems and chronic pain. It highlights so very well that "life isn't about waiting for the storm to pass, it's about learning to be and dance in the rain".

Mindfulness for Health offers those who struggle with the painful loss of health much support to become more alive and compassionate and not trapped by pain and ill health. This truly resourceful book will help people grow their own sense of self and a new more rewarding life, and lessen their suffering. Readers will want to touch and refresh its kindly guidance every day'

Dr Frances Cole, GP
Pain Rehabilitation Specialist and CBT therapist
Leeds Community Trust Spinal Pain Management Service, UK

'Vidyamala and Danny have demonstrated their compassion and ability to teach mindfulness from the inside out in this book. The programme detailed is transparent and user-friendly. Thoughtful and practical strategies are offered for those with pain. For health professionals assisting those with ill-health, it intuitively re-orders the guiding of the development of a mindfulness practice and boldly integrates compassion. This will be an important resource for the mindfulness community'

Dr Elizabeth Foley
Senior MBCT Facilitator & Researcher
Sydney, Australia

'Living with pain, illness and stress is challenging. Through a lens of kindness, compassion and acceptance Vidyamala Burch and Danny

Penman bring a softer focus to pain and suffering. Drawing on personal experience and wise counsel, they guide the reader through practical and proven techniques to empower and support them through their journey to wholeness and healing. They show how the benefits of mindfulness can bring a different kind of healing so that the mind–body can be calmed, focused, refreshed and renewed'

Liz Lobb
Professor of Palliative Care, Sydney, Australia

'The appealing thing about mindfulness is that it is a technique you can learn yourself and practise to continuously enhance your own health. The distress of persistent pain often drives us to repeatedly seek escape and control through medication, interventions and therapies. Yet for many of us, pain remains the dominant part of our lives. Mindfulness offers a distinctly compassionate and authentic way to reconcile our experiences of pain. Vidyamala Burch and Danny Penman have set out a humane and accessible pathway to bring mindfulness into a daily routine. I would really encourage you to give yourself eight weeks with this book. You will be rewarded with a profound change'

Dr Margaret Macky, FAFOEM
Occupational Medicine Specialist, New Zealand

'Meeting pain with the "tender gravity of kindness" is courageous and transformative. Vidyamala Burch and Danny Penman "walk the talk"; they invite people suffering pain to reclaim their lives through this accessible, personal, wise and eminently commonsensical guide'

Willem Kuyken
Professor of Clinical Psychology, University of Exeter

Mindfulness for Health

a practical guide to

RELIEVING PAIN, REDUCING STRESS AND RESTORING WELLBEING

VIDYAMALA BURCH and DANNY PENMAN,

co-author of the bestselling *Mindfulness*

FOREWORD BY MARK WILLIAMS

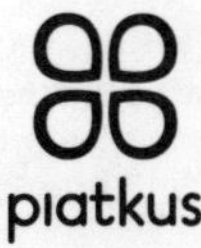

PIATKUS

First published in Great Britain in 2013 by Piatkus

10

A CIP catalogue record for this book is available from the British Library.

ISBN 978-0-7499-5924-1

Typeset in Sabon by M Rules
Printed and bound in Great Britain by
Clays Ltd, St Ives plc

Papers used by Piatkus are from well-managed forests and other responsible sources.

Piatkus
An imprint of
Little, Brown Book Group
Carmelite House
50 Victoria Embankment
London EC4Y 0DZ

An Hachette UK Company
www.hachette.co.uk

www.littlebrown.co.uk

Please take responsibility for your own body. Seek advice from your health professional if you have doubts about any aspect of the programme. If you already have a physiotherapy or exercise plan that works for you, then keep doing it alongside this one. Meditation is not a substitute for medication. Please do not alter any of the medicines that you take without first consulting your health professional. You may well find that you can reduce your dose, but make sure this is done gradually and is well managed. Even if you find you can't reduce your medication, mindfulness will still help you to get your life back on track by bringing a new richness and texture to your days.

There is a variety of ways in which to support your learning when completing the course in this book. Through Breathworks, you can do it in a group with others or join an online group. Individual tuition and support are also available (for more details and a list of accredited Breathworks trainers visit www.breathworks-mindfulness.org.uk).

DEDICATION

For sweet little Sasha May Penman

Danny

For everyone at Breathworks – with deep gratitude for sharing my vision and making it real

Vidyamala

CONTENTS

ACKNOWLEDGEMENTS

This book could not have been written without a diverse network of people who generously gave their time, help and support throughout.

We are enormously grateful to Sheila Crowley at Curtis Brown and to Anne Lawrance and her team at Piatkus. Vidyamala is especially grateful to the UK's Millennium Commission, which in 2001 awarded her a grant for disabled people who wished to contribute to the community. Without this initial input, the 'Peace of Mind' project would not have been created and Breathworks, as the project became known in 2004, would never have come into being. Special thanks must also go to Breathworks co-founders Sona Fricker and Gary Hennessey, along with the rest of the core team based in Manchester: Colin Duff, Singhashri Gazmuri, Jennifer Jones, Di Kaylor and Karunavajri Morris. We are also grateful to the hundreds of trainers working worldwide who are dedicated to sharing the Breathworks message, as well as the thousands of people who are ill and living with pain who have involved themselves in

Breathworks over the years. Their courage and openness have helped us formulate the material in this book. Over the years, many of these people have generously shared their stories with us. When they are included in this book, we've changed their names to protect their privacy.

The main content of the programme in this book is based on an online course written by Vidyamala and developed in conjunction with the Mindfulness Center in Sweden, founded by Dr Ola Schenstrom.

Danny is especially grateful to Mr Mark Jackson and his team at the Bristol Royal Infirmary who reconstructed his leg following a paragliding accident. This incident led him to begin using mindfulness for pain relief and to speed healing.

Thanks also to our team of academic and medical advisers, all of whom have dedicated many years to helping people manage the suffering associated with chronic pain: Professor Lance McCracken of King's College and St Thomas' NHS Foundation Trust; Professor Stephen Morley of the University of Leeds; and Dr Amanda C de C Williams of University College London.

We are especially grateful to Jon Kabat-Zinn, the pioneering scientist at the University of Massachusetts Medical Center who brought mindfulness to Western healthcare. And, of course, a warm and grateful thanks must go to Professor Mark Williams of Oxford University, who has always been a great supporter of our work.

Thanks also to Sona, Vidyamala's partner, and to Bella, Danny's wife, who gave their tireless support. And Danny's baby daughter, Sasha May, has been an inspiration throughout.

FOREWORD BY MARK WILLIAMS

There is a curious paradox at the heart of mindfulness training. Mindfulness means 'awareness', yet surely when any of us are suffering from the searing physical pain that may arise with a chronic illness or traumatic injury, we seem to be *too* aware of our suffering. How on earth can learning to become even *more* aware possibly help?

Vidyamala Burch and Danny Penman explain how, in this beautiful and compassionate book. They describe how certain very subtle processes of mind can switch on automatically to turn up the volume on the very pain and discomfort you want to get rid of. It is because these aggravating factors switch on automatically, without your awareness, that the spotlight of attention is needed. If it all happens 'in the dark', you remain lost and alone with your pain. But if you can shine the light of attention upon your suffering, then it begins to dissolve.

But Vidyamala and Danny don't just give a clear and up-to-date scientific explanation of how this happens; they also provide a step-by-step guide to help you through your suffering. At the heart of this is a series of short meditation practices that will build the courage to enable you to move in closer to the centre of the intensity, to investigate it with friendliness and curiosity, so you can begin to see more clearly where the automatic tendencies of the mind begin to take over. They show how you can discern which activities help or harm you, and how to 'incline the mind', which is often harsh and unforgiving, towards an openness and compassion that, strange as it may seem, dissolves much of the suffering that once seemed so inevitable.

I have been privileged to know both Vidyamala and Danny for many years. Both write from their own experience: each knows what it is like to suffer pain that seemed to them, at one time, unendurable. For Vidyamala, it was as a result of a lifting accident followed by a road traffic accident five years later; for Danny it was due to a paragliding accident. They describe these experiences in the book, and how they found themselves trapped in both acute and chronic pain from which there seemed no escape. Both found, in the cultivation of mindfulness meditation, a path to freedom from their suffering. On the basis of her experience, Vidyamala wrote *Living Well with Pain and Illness*, and founded Breathworks, an organisation to help those who suffer from chronic pain, illness and stress. She has helped countless people through her writing and her clinical and training work. On the basis of his experience, Danny discovered Mindfulness-Based Cognitive Therapy (MBCT), and wrote about it eloquently in the bestseller *Mindfulness: a practical guide to finding peace in a frantic world* – a book that has been a help to many.

The book you hold in your hands contains many inspiring stories from people who had given up all hope, whose lives seemed irreversibly damaged by their illness, accident or trauma. For some of those featured, the encouragement provided by the modern scientific understandings of pain – and the evidence that mindfulness can provide a radically new and effective approach to such suffering – may have inspired them to participate in mindfulness classes. But while science can motivate the first move, it is less likely to sustain that motivation when things get really tough. It is at this point that the underlying philosophy of mindfulness, and of the originator of its use in the modern healthcare system, Jon Kabat-Zinn, comes into its own. He has said that, no matter what illnesses and injuries you are carrying, while you are still breathing there is more right with you than wrong with you.

With this understanding of illness, the mindful approach to mind–body medicine is to see everyone as having deep resources that they are unaware of because no one has told them how to recognise and cultivate them. The pain cannot be ignored or wished away. But underneath the clanging noise of the pain there is a deep wholeness that cannot be damaged by illness and disease, a wholeness that can be re-inhabited if, just for a moment, we could approach willingly, sense precisely and befriend tenderly the body that seems to be letting us down so badly.

Cultivating this approach is not easy, but it is doable. It takes patience, courage and a willingness to do the work of practice. No one else can do this work for you, but good and trustworthy guides are invaluable. Vidyamala and Danny have written this book to guide you through the process. May their guidance allow you to discover the profound benefits of mindfulness, as the practice day by day gradually puts you back in touch with the extraordinary person you already are.

Professor Mark Williams
University of Oxford

CHAPTER ONE

Every Moment is a New Chance

Pain always seems worse at night. There is something about the silence that amplifies the suffering. Even after you've taken the maximum dose of painkillers, the aching soon returns with a vengeance. You want to do something, *anything*, to stop the pain, but whatever you try seems to fail. Moving hurts. Doing nothing hurts. Ignoring it hurts. But it's not just the pain that hurts; your mind can start to suffer as you desperately try to find a way of escaping. Pointed and bitter questions can begin nagging at your soul: *What will happen if I don't recover? What if it gets worse? I can't cope with this ... Please, I just want it to stop ...*

We wrote this book to help you cope with pain, illness and stress in times such as these. It will teach you how to reduce your suffering progressively, so that you can begin living life to the full once again. It may not completely eliminate your suffering, but it will ensure that it no longer dominates your life. You'll discover that it *is* possible to be at peace, even if illness and pain are unavoidable, and to enjoy a truly fulfilling life.

We know this to be true because we have both experienced terrible injuries and used an ancient form of meditation known as 'mindfulness' to ease our suffering. The techniques in this book have been proven to work by doctors and scientists in universities around the world. In fact, mindfulness is so effective that doctors and specialist pain clinics now refer their patients to our Breathworks centre in Manchester and to courses run by our affiliated trainers around the world. Every day we help people find peace amid their suffering.

This book and the accompanying CD reveal a series of simple practices that you can incorporate into daily life to significantly reduce your pain, anguish and stress.[1] They are built on Mindfulness-Based Pain Management (MBPM), which has its roots in the ground-breaking work of Dr Jon Kabat-Zinn of the University of Massachusetts Medical Center in America. The MBPM programme itself was developed by Vidyamala Burch (co-author of this book) as a means of coping with the after-effects of two serious accidents. Although originally designed to reduce physical pain and suffering, it has proven to be an effective stress-reduction technique as well. In fact, the core mindfulness meditation techniques have been shown in many clinical trials to be at least as effective as drugs or counselling for relieving anxiety, stress and depression.[2] When it comes to pain, clinical trials show that mindfulness can be as effective as the main prescription painkillers, and some studies have shown it to be as powerful as morphine. Imaging studies show that it soothes the brain patterns underlying pain and, over time, these changes take root and alter the structure of the brain itself so that you no longer feel pain with the same intensity. And when it does arise, the pain no longer dominates your life so much.[3,4] Many people report that their pain declines to such a degree that they barely notice it at all.

Many hospital pain clinics now prescribe mindfulness meditation to help patients cope with the suffering arising from a wide range of diseases such as cancer (and the side effects of chemotherapy), heart disease, diabetes and arthritis. It is also used for back problems, migraine, fibromyalgia, coeliac disease, and a range of auto-immune diseases such as lupus and multiple sclerosis, as well as being effective for such long-term conditions as chronic fatigue syndrome and irritable bowel syndrome. It's also useful for coping with labour pain. In addition to all these uses, clinical trials also show that mindfulness significantly reduces the anxiety, stress, depression, irritability and insomnia that can arise from chronic pain and illness. Researchers are continually finding new conditions that can be eased with mindfulness.

The benefits of mindfulness meditation

Thousands of peer-reviewed scientific papers prove that mindfulness reduces pain, enhances mental and physical wellbeing and helps people deal with the stresses and strains of daily life. Here are a few of the main findings:

- Mindfulness can dramatically reduce pain and the emotional reaction to it.[5,6] Recent trials suggest that average pain 'unpleasantness' levels can be reduced by 57 per cent while accomplished meditators report reductions of up to 93 per cent.[7]

- Clinical trials show that mindfulness improves mood and quality of life in chronic pain conditions such as fibromyalgia[8] and lower-back pain,[9] in chronic functional disorders such as IBS,[10] and in challenging medical illnesses, including multiple sclerosis[11] and cancer.[12]
- Mindfulness improves working memory, creativity, attention span and reaction speeds. It also enhances mental and physical stamina and resilience.[13]
- Meditation improves emotional intelligence.[14]
- Mindfulness is a potent antidote to anxiety, stress, depression, exhaustion and irritability. In short, regular meditators are happier and more contented, while being far less likely to suffer from psychological distress.[15]
- Mindfulness is at least as good as drugs or counselling for the treatment of clinical-level depression. One structured programme known as Mindfulness-Based Cognitive Therapy (MBCT) is now one of the preferred treatments recommended by the UK's National Institute for Health and Clinical Excellence.[16]
- Mindfulness reduces addictive and self-destructive behaviour. These include the abuse of illegal and prescription drugs and excessive alcohol intake.[17]
- Meditation enhances brain function. It increases grey matter in areas associated with self-awareness, empathy, self-control and

attention.[18] It soothes the parts of the brain that produce stress hormones[19] and builds those areas that lift mood and promote learning.[20] It even reduces some of the thinning of certain areas of the brain that naturally occurs with ageing.[21]

- Meditation improves the immune system. Regular meditators are admitted to hospital far less often for cancer, heart disease and numerous infectious diseases.[22]
- Mindfulness may reduce ageing at the cellular level by promoting chromosomal health and resilience.[23]
- Meditation and mindfulness improve control of blood sugar in type II diabetes.[24]
- Meditation improves heart and circulatory health by reducing blood pressure and lowering the risk of hypertension. Mindfulness reduces the risks of developing and dying from cardiovascular disease and lowers its severity should it arise.[25]

MINDFULNESS DISSOLVES PAIN AND SUFFERING

Mindfulness-Based Pain Management uses ancient meditations that were largely unknown in the West until recently. A typical meditation involves focusing on the breath as it flows into and out of the body (see box on page 9). This allows you to see your mind and body in action, to observe painful sensations as they arise and to let go of struggling with them. Mindfulness teaches you that pain naturally waxes and wanes. You learn to gently observe it, rather than be caught up in it, and when you do so, something remarkable happens: it begins to melt away of its own accord. After a while you come to the profound realisation that pain comes in two forms: Primary and Secondary. Each of these has very different causes – and understanding this gives you far greater control over your suffering.

Primary pain tends to arise from illness, injury or damage to the body or nervous system. You could see it as raw information being sent by the body to the brain. Secondary pain follows on close behind, but is often far more powerful and distressing. Secondary pain can be seen as the mind's reaction to Primary pain.

Pain's volume control

The mind has tremendous control over the sensations of pain that you consciously feel and how unpleasant they are.[26] It has a 'volume' control that governs both the intensity and duration of the sensations of pain. This is because your mind does not simply feel pain, it also processes the information that it contains. It teases apart all of the different sensations to try to find their underlying causes so that you can avoid further pain or damage to the body. In effect, your mind zooms in on your pain for a closer look as it tries to find a solution to your suffering. This 'zooming-in' amplifies your pain. As your mind analyses the pain, it also sifts through your memories for occasions when you have suffered similarly in the past. It is searching for a pattern, some clues, that will lead to a solution. Trouble is, if you have suffered from pain or illness for months or years, then the mind will have a rich tapestry of painful memories on which to draw – but very few solutions. So before you know it, your mind can become flooded with unsettling memories. You can become enmeshed in thoughts about your suffering. It can seem as if you've always been ill and in pain, that you've never found a solution and that you never will. So you can end up being consumed by future anxieties, stresses and worries as well as physical pain: *What will happen if I can't stop this pain? Am I going to spend my life suffering like this? Is it going to keep on getting worse?*

This process happens in an instant, before you're consciously aware of it. Each thought builds on the last and quickly turns into a vicious cycle that ends up further amplifying your pain. And it can be worse than this because such stresses and fears feed back into the body to create even more tension and stress. This can aggravate illnesses and injuries, leading to even more pain. It also dampens down the immune system, so impairing healing. So you can all too easily become trapped in a vicious downward spiral that leads to ever greater suffering.

But even worse, such negative spirals can begin wearing tracks in the mind so that you become primed to suffer. Your brain begins fine-tuning itself to sense pain more quickly – and with greater intensity – in a futile bid to try to avoid the worst of it. Over time, the brain actually becomes *better* at sensing pain. Brain scans confirm that people who suffer from chronic pain have more brain tissue dedicated to feeling the conscious sensations of pain.[27] It's almost as if the brain has turned up the volume to maximum and doesn't know how to turn it down again.

It's important to emphasise that Secondary pain is *real*. You do genuinely feel it. It's only called Secondary pain because it is the mind's reaction to Primary pain and has been heavily processed before you consciously feel it. But this same processing also gives you a way out; it means you can learn to gain control over your pain. For this reason, Secondary pain is best described as *suffering*.

In practice, you can be in pain but you need not *suffer*.

Once you realise this, deep in your heart, then you can learn to step aside from your suffering and begin to handle pain very differently indeed. In effect, mindfulness hands back to you the volume control for your pain.

The benefits of mindfulness on overall mental and physical health have been demonstrated in a wide range of scientific studies. Despite this, you might still be a little sceptical about meditation.[28] When the word is mentioned a whole cascade of stereotypes can spring to mind: Buddhist monks, yoga classes, lentils, brown rice . . . So, before we proceed, we'd like to dispel some myths:

- Meditation is not a religion. It is simply a form of mental training that has been proven in countless scientific trials to help people cope with pain, illness, anxiety, stress, depression, irritability and exhaustion.

- Meditation will not trick you into passivity or resign you to your fate. On the contrary, mindfulness boosts mental and physical resilience.

- Meditation will not seduce you into adopting a fake 'positive' attitude to life. It simply creates a form of mental clarity that helps you to enjoy life and achieve your goals.

- Meditation does not take a lot of time. The programme in this book takes around twenty minutes per day. In fact, many people find that it liberates more time than it consumes because they spend far less time having to cope with chronic pain, illness and stress.

- Meditation is not difficult or complicated, although it does require some effort and persistence. You can meditate on more or less anything (see the Coffee Meditation in Chapter Three). You can also do it virtually anywhere – on buses, trains, aircraft or even in the busiest office.

A simple breath-based meditation

Meditation can be simple and does not require any special equipment. The meditation below demonstrates the basic technique and takes just a few minutes. It will leave you profoundly relaxed.

1. If your condition allows it, sit erect but relaxed in a straight-backed chair with your feet flat on the floor. If you cannot sit, then lie on a mat or blanket on the floor, or on your bed. Allow your arms and hands to be as relaxed as possible.
2. Gently close your eyes and focus your awareness on the breath as it flows into and out of your body. Feel the sensations the air makes as it flows in through your mouth or nose, down your throat and into your lungs. Feel the expansion and subsiding of your chest and belly as you breathe. Focus your awareness on where the sensations are strongest. Stay in contact with each in-breath and each out-breath. Observe it without trying to alter it in any way or expecting anything special to happen.

3. When your mind wanders, gently shepherd it back to the breath. Try not to criticise yourself. Minds wander. It's what they do. The act of realising that your mind has wandered – and encouraging it to return to focus on the breath – is central to the practice of mindfulness.

4. Your mind may eventually become calm – or it may not. If it becomes calm, then this may only be short-lived. Your mind may become filled with thoughts or powerful emotions such as fear, anger, stress or love. These may also be fleeting. Whatever happens, simply observe as best you can without reacting to your experience or trying to change anything. Gently return your awareness back to the sensations of the breath again and again.

5. After a few minutes, or longer if you prefer, gently open your eyes and take in your surroundings.

MINDFULNESS FOR HEALTH

This book operates on two levels, which unfold week by week. The core mindfulness programme takes eight weeks and there is a chapter dedicated to each step. Each week you'll be asked to carry out two meditations on six days out of seven. These take just ten minutes each.

You'll also be encouraged to break some of your unconscious habits of thinking and behaving. These can embed a surprising amount of suffering because much of what we think and feel is locked in place by ongoing ways of approaching the world. By simply breaking some of your more ingrained habits you will help dissolve away your suffering. Habit-breaking – we prefer the term 'habit-releasing' – is straightforward. It can be as simple as watching the clouds from a park bench or waiting for the kettle to fully boil before making a cup of tea or coffee (rather than rushing to switch it off).

The programme in this book is best carried out over the recommended eight weeks, although you can do it over a longer period if you wish. Many people find that mindfulness gives them so many benefits that they continue with it for the rest of their lives. They see it as a journey that continuously reveals their true potential.

It can be a long and fruitful journey. We wish you well.

The next chapter explains the science behind mindfulness and how it dissolves pain, suffering and stress, and restores wellbeing. Reading it will improve the effectiveness of the whole programme. If you wish to begin the programme immediately, feel free to do so, but try to come back to Chapter Two when you get the chance. It really does enhance the whole experience.

The accompanying CD, recorded by Vidyamala, contains the meditation tracks that you will need to carry out the programme. For best results, we suggest that you first read through the meditations found in each of the eight practice chapters to familiarise yourself with what's required. Then, it is best if you carry out the actual meditations while listening to the corresponding tracks. You can also download these as MP3 files via: www.franticworld.com/health or http://www.breathworks-mindfulness.org.uk/health

Note: you will need an up-to-date browser in order to download the files.

CHAPTER TWO

What You Resist Persists

Claire stared at the computer screen before cocking her head slightly to one side. She winced as a sharp pain angled its way through her neck and down her left arm. Her fingers went numb and then began to throb. Claire's youthful good looks dissolved and she suddenly looked twenty years older. She stretched her arm and slowly began rubbing her neck to loosen the muscles. Her shoulders and neck had cramped up, making her whole upper body look tense and contorted. She reached for a glass of water and gulped down two more painkillers.

Why won't this pain just stop? Why won't these blasted painkillers work any more? They're useless. I'm so sick and tired of this.

Three years previously Claire had been injured in a car crash and suffered two broken ribs, a fractured wrist and whiplash. Her ribs and wrist had healed completely within three months, but the after-effects of her whiplash refused to go away. The doctors were puzzled by her pain. Several scans had shown that her neck had completely healed, but the pain stubbornly remained. It was worse if she stayed in one place for too long. After twenty minutes, sharp jagged pains would arc up and down her neck. When she finally did move, she would feel stiff and achy all over.

Claire felt increasingly trapped and broken. Her doctor had prescribed several courses of physiotherapy without any long-term success. Now she was forced to continually take painkillers and anti-inflammatory drugs. They worked, more or less, but often left her feeling washed out and jaded. They were OK for stubborn 'achiness', but did nothing for the frequent sharp twinges of pain. Lately, her doctor had begun suggesting antidepressants to lift her mood. Her response was always the same: 'I'm not depressed,' she'd snap. 'I'm *angry* because that man who drove into me has taken my life away. I used to dance all night. Now I can barely walk!'

Experiences like Claire's are not confined to injuries such as whiplash, but are common across a range of diseases. Conditions such as 'bad back', migraine, chronic fatigue syndrome and fibromyalgia can all cause pain long after the original injuries have healed or without any obvious cause that shows up on scans or tests. And even when there is a clear physical cause, as with illnesses like arthritis, heart disease or cancer, the pain often comes and goes without any apparent rhyme or reason. Doctors then feel forced to prescribe long-term courses of painkillers, but these can have side effects such as memory loss, lethargy and even addiction.

Claire and millions of others exist in a world of suffering; a place where even the simplest of tasks can amplify their pain. This often leads to anxiety, stress, depression and exhaustion, each of which serves to further enhance suffering in a downward spiral. Such vicious cycles are driven by newly discovered psychological forces that underlie the perception of pain. And crucially, this discovery offers a wholly new approach to the management of pain and illness that has the potential to transform suffering. It is important to understand these underlying forces because such knowledge enhances the effectiveness of the whole mindfulness programme.

WHAT IS PAIN?

The commonsense view of pain is that it arises from damage to the body. This attitude was formalised in the seventeenth century by the French philosopher René Descartes with his 'rope-pull' model of pain: just as pulling a rope in a church steeple rings a bell, Descartes thought that damage to the body is a tug that causes the awareness of pain in the brain. For centuries after Descartes, doctors regarded pain in a similar light. The intensity of pain was thought to be directly proportional to the degree of damage to the body, which would mean that if different people had the same injury they would experience the same amount of pain. If no obvious physical cause was found, the patient would be regarded as malingering or making it up.

Since the 1960s, science has come to accept another model of pain known as the 'Gate Theory' developed by Ronald Melzack and Patrick Wall.[1] They suggest that there are 'gates' in the brain and nervous system that, when open, allow you to experience pain. In a sense, the body sends a continuous low-level 'chatter' of pain signals to the brain, but it is only when the gates are opened that the signals reach your conscious mind. These gates can also close, which is what happens when your pain lessens or fades away.

Opening and closing these pain gates is a phenomenally complex process. Although the details are still being worked out, it is clear that pain is far more subtle and complex than the traditional idea of damage signals being sent to the brain which are then passively felt. Pain is a *sensation,* which means that it is an interpretation made by the brain before it is consciously felt. To make this interpretation, the brain fuses together information from the *mind* as well as the body. In practice, this means that the thoughts and emotions flowing through your mind, both conscious and unconscious, have a dramatic effect on the intensity of your suffering. Not without reason did the ancient Greek philosophers consider pain to be an emotion.

The many faces of pain

Acute pain occurs in the short term and is usually a direct response to an injury. It's part of the body's inbuilt alarm system, signalling that it's under attack and that you should take care of the injured area. It normally leads to inflammation such as a bruise or swelling. Most healing is completed within six weeks and acute pain usually reduces over this period. Nearly all injured tissues are fully healed within six months. Acute pain also arises without obvious injury, as with a stomachache after overeating, or the headache that comes with a hangover.

Chronic pain is the type that lasts for three months or more.[2] The word 'chronic' is often misunderstood to mean 'severe', but what it actually means is 'long-term'. It sometimes develops after an injury and persists, often inexplicably, even after tissue healing has taken place. Some chronic pain is caused by damage that persists over time; this is the case, for example, with arthritis and cancer. Chronic pain may also start for no obvious or specific reason. If the pain remains when there's no continuing physical damage, it becomes a medical problem in its own right and is often known as 'chronic pain syndrome'.

Neuropathic pain occurs in the nervous system and often normal investigations fail to discover a clear cause. It might result from damage to the nerves, spinal cord or brain. But sometimes pain is felt even when there is no damage, or when healing seems to have completed at the site of an illness or injury. One possibility is that background 'noise' in the nervous system becomes unduly amplified. This is believed to happen because the nervous system responds to the experience of pain by increasing its capacity to process pain signals – rather as a computer devotes extra memory and circuits to an important task. So it begins to act like an amplifier that's stuck on 'high'. Neuropathic pain can also take the form of unusual sensations, such as burning, electric shocks and can even 'occur' in amputated limbs. Some forms of tinnitus (ringing or 'white noise' sounds in the ears) can be considered to be neuropathic pain.

PRIMARY AND SECONDARY SUFFERING

Suffering occurs on two levels. Firstly, there are the actual unpleasant sensations felt in the body – this is known as 'Primary Suffering'. This can be seen as the 'raw data' that is sent to the brain from, say, an injury, an ongoing illness or changes to the nervous system itself (this is believed to lie, at least partly, behind such conditions as chronic pain syndrome and phantom limb syndrome). Overlaid on top of this is 'Secondary Suffering', which is made up of all the thoughts, feelings, emotions and memories associated with the pain. These might include anxiety, stress, worry, depression and feelings of hopelessness and exhaustion. The pain and distress that you *actually* feel is a fusion of both Primary and Secondary Suffering.

This insight is crucial because it reveals a path away from suffering. For if you can learn to tease apart the two flavours of suffering, you can greatly reduce – or even eliminate – your pain and distress. This is because Secondary Suffering tends to dissolve when you observe it with the mind's compassionate eye. Mindfulness allows you to see the different elements of pain laid out in front of you. And when you see this vista, something remarkable begins to happen: your suffering gradually begins to subside and evaporate like the mist on a summer's morning.

It's important to understand that although the sensation of pain is created by the mind, your suffering is still real. You really *do* feel it. It exists and it can be genuinely overwhelming. But once you understand the underlying mechanisms of pain, you can begin to temper its power and the hold it has over you.

Pain and Suffering

Chronic pain is becoming increasingly common and exacts a staggering toll on society. On average, around one in five people in the developed world now suffers from chronic pain, and a recent survey in the UK reported that 31 per cent of men and 37 per cent of women experience it.[3] This equates to around 20 million people in the UK with 7.8 million of them suffering moderate to severe pain that has lasted for more than six months. Figures are similar in the USA with some 116 million people suffering chronic pain causing estimated costs of $635 billion a year, which is more than the yearly costs for cancer, heart disease and diabetes.[4] And the problem is likely to become worse as an ageing population begins to suffer increasing infirmity. Already, half of the over-seventy-fives suffer pain on a daily basis.[5] Increasing levels of obesity and a sedentary lifestyle will add to the problem as they increase wear and tear on the body.

The biggest causes of chronic pain are back problems, arthritis, injury and headaches. Following close behind are conditions such as cancer (and its associated chemotherapy), heart disease, fibromyalgia, coeliac disease, lupus, chronic fatigue syndrome and irritable bowel syndrome.

If all this wasn't bad enough, chronic pain can lead to clinical-level anxiety, stress, depression, irritability, anger and exhaustion. A survey for the British Pain Society, for example, found that half of those with chronic pain subsequently suffered from depression.[6] Given that mental-health problems are increasing across society, within a few decades the default human condition will become one of chronic pain, anxiety, stress and depression, rather than being characterised by quiet contentment and happiness.

To go back to Claire, had she been asked to look inside herself a little more closely she would have realised that there was not one single 'thing' that she could label as an 'ache' or as a 'pain'. Both were 'bundles' of different feelings that were constantly changing;

becoming either more or less intense. There was the underlying unpleasant 'tightness' of the muscles and tendons in her neck, which were twisting her vertebrae slightly out of alignment and creating the most pronounced of her painful feelings. There were also twinges of outright pain – which felt like sharp spikes of electricity running through her muscles and down into her arm. And then there were patches of 'numbness' in her left arm and hand. These would alternate with pins and needles. Those were the obvious sensations of pain. This was her Primary Suffering.

But there were other feelings too – powerful emotions and disturbing thoughts that would frequently sweep across her mind, often with no apparent rhyme or reason. Stress, worry and exhaustion had become a way of life. Troubling thoughts constantly nagged at her soul: *Why won't this just stop? The doctors must have missed something, surely? Maybe I'm going to end up a cripple, or even dead. Are they too afraid to tell me?* Such thoughts and emotions were constantly bubbling away in the background. And while they were often less obvious than the nagging feelings of pain, ultimately they were far more significant because they were central to the way that her mind interpreted and felt the raw feelings of pain. In a sense, they controlled the intensity or 'volume' of her pain. This was Secondary Suffering; and Claire had it in spades.

Claire's Secondary Suffering had its roots in the five days she spent in hospital after her accident. They were the worst of her life. She was in considerable pain and on a morphine drip for the first twenty-four hours. She could cope with the physical pain – just. Far worse, however, were her turbulent emotions: her fears and worries for herself and the future. Neither she nor the doctors could predict the outcome of her neck injuries. Would she be partially paralysed? Would she be in pain for the rest of her life? There was also a sense of anger mixed with bitterness. The man who crashed into her didn't appear to care. He just walked away from the accident with no cuts or bruises at all. He'd been drinking, but was just inside the legal drink–drive limit. Was he insured? It turned out he wasn't. Every time she thought about it, Claire's anger boiled over. Such thoughts and overwhelming emotions constantly washed across her mind. It was mental pain and just as real and tormenting as her physical injuries.

She lay in her hospital bed at night crying quietly to herself. She was wracked with fears and worries for the future, and 'what ifs' filled her mind. If only she had left home a minute or two later, then none of it would have happened. She'd had a feeling something was wrong before she had left home. Why hadn't she waited just a few minutes longer?

After the accident and the subsequent months of physiotherapy, a new emotion was added to the list: depression. Claire refused to believe that she was depressed, but it was there none the less, gnawing away at her in the background. It wasn't an all-consuming depression. It simply drained her of all energy and enthusiasm for life. Such powerful emotions as anxiety, fear, anger, worry and depression can feed into the mind's perception of pain. Other feelings, too, can have an incredibly strong effect. Feeling tired and overwhelmed, fragile and broken, stressed and anxious, can all magnify suffering and tip you into a downward spiral. How often has the intensity of your suffering increased when you felt anxious, stressed, exhausted or sad? These emotions act like amplifiers in the mind's pain circuits. They can open the floodgates of suffering.

The effect of such emotions can be observed with a brain scanner. Work at Oxford University,[7] for example, shows the significant impact that even mild levels of anxiety can have on pain. Scientists at the university's Department of Clinical Neurology induced low-level anxiety in a group of volunteers before burning the back of their left hand with a hot probe. As anxiety built, you could see the waves of emotion sweeping through the volunteers' brains. This primed areas of the brain that collectively make up the 'pain matrix'. It was almost as if the volunteers' minds were turning up the volume on their pain amplifiers ready to 'hear' its first 'notes', so that they could take action to protect themselves. This meant that when the skin of the anxious volunteers was actually burned, they experienced far more pain and suffering than the 'non-anxious' volunteers. You could see this extra pain represented in the brain scans too. As the Oxford neuroscientists noted, anxiety primes the 'behavioural responses that are adaptive to the worst possible outcome'. In other words, anxiety and other powerful 'negative' emotions prepare the body to sense pain quickly and with great intensity.

The reverse is also true. Reducing anxiety, stress, depression and exhaustion can lower the perception of pain and even eliminate it completely. This is one of the main routes by which mindfulness helps reduce suffering. Mindfulness soothes the mind's perception of pain – essentially Secondary Suffering – by replacing it with a sense of peace and wholeness.

Neuroscientist Fadel Zeidan and his team at Wake Forest University School of Medicine in America decided to investigate this effect using scanners to map activity in different parts of the brain.[8] They did this by exploiting a curious quirk of brain anatomy. Every part of the body is reflected in a specific part of the brain known as the primary somatosensory cortex. So if the sole of your left foot is brushed with a feather, an area of the primary somatosensory cortex lights up; if you feel a pain in your lower back, a different part becomes active. Neurosurgeon Wilder Penfield charted this brain region and produced a 'map' that reflects the human body overlaid on the brain (see illustration below). It was termed the cortical 'homunculus'.

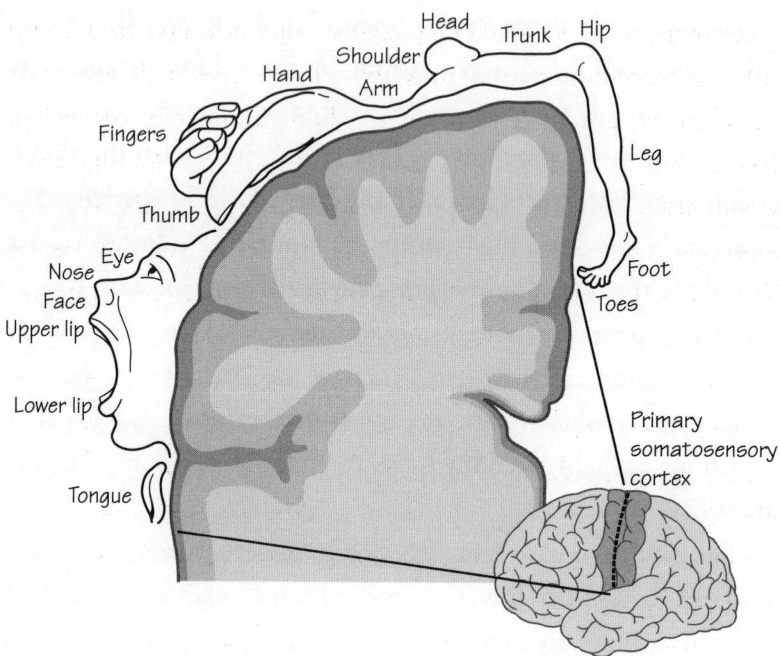

Fadel Zeidan and his team reasoned that if mindfulness affected the perception of pain, then this should be visibly reflected in the level of activity in the corresponding regions of the primary somatosensory cortex. To test this, Zeidan studied the perception of pain in a group of students. The students first had the back of their right calf burned with a piece of hot metal while their brain was scanned with the latest functional Magnetic Resonance Imaging (fMRI) scanner. Each was then asked to rate both the intensity and unpleasantness of the pain.

If pain was music, 'intensity' would be the volume and 'unpleasantness' would be the level of emotion it aroused. As expected, when the students' legs were burned the 'right calf' region of their primary somatosensory cortex lit up as the pain swept over them.

The students were then taught mindfulness meditation and the experiment was repeated. The results could not have been more different second time around. Activity in the 'right calf' region of the primary somatosensory cortex had diminished to such a degree that it had become undetectable. But not only that. Meditation increased activity in regions of the brain related to the processing of emotion and of cognitive control – areas where the sensations of pain are actually interpreted and 'built'. These brain areas modulate the sensations of pain and give it 'meaning' before it is consciously felt. What's more, experienced meditators (those who scored higher on a standard scale of mindfulness) tended to have enhanced activity in these regions and to experience less pain. That is, they tended to devote more brain power in this region to moderating the pain-related information – and to, in effect, turning down its 'volume'.

Zeidan's co-worker Dr Robert C. Coghill explains:

> These areas all shape how the brain builds an experience of pain from nerve signals that are coming in from the body. Consistent with this function, the more that these areas were activated by meditation, the more that pain was reduced. One of the reasons that meditation may have been so effective in blocking pain was that it did not work at just one place in the brain, but instead reduced pain at multiple levels of processing.

And what of the students' conscious experience of pain? On average they experienced a 40 per cent reduction in pain intensity and a 57 per cent lessening of pain 'unpleasantness'. Perhaps the most surprising thing was the amount of practice required to achieve this level of pain relief: just four training sessions of twenty minutes each.

Remarkable though these results were, they masked something even more intriguing. The more accomplished meditators suffered far less than these averages might suggest. They experienced a reduction in pain intensity of 70 per cent and its unpleasantness was reduced by 93 per cent. This meant that it could barely be felt and hardly bothered them at all. Overall, said Zeidan, mindfulness produced a greater reduction in pain than standard doses of morphine and other pain-relieving drugs.

Loosening the bonds of pain

Secondary Suffering can be seen as resistance to pain. It is entirely natural to struggle against and resist pain with all of your might. You want to eliminate it. Stamp on it. Do anything at all to get rid of it. This is absolutely understandable. But what if this was also precisely the wrong approach? What if, in your bid to eliminate pain, you were actually creating far more of it instead? This is the lesson from Zeidan's research and from many other studies too. And this holds true not just for pain, but for many other disease symptoms as well. Stress, exhaustion and depression can all be made far worse through resistance.

But if the act of resisting pain can make it worse, the converse is also true. Acceptance of your pain can actually diminish it – and might even get rid of it completely. Allow us to explain this seemingly outrageous idea.

Neuroscientists have a saying: 'What we resist persists.' In other words, if you resist the messages that your mind and body are sending you, those messages will keep on being dispatched (and felt) until you accept them. This holds true not only for messages of pain, but also for thoughts, feelings, emotions, memories and judgements. If you mindfully accept (or feel) these messages, they will have done their job and will tend to melt away of their own accord.

Mindfulness meditation creates a sense of safety, of space, in which you can begin to tentatively explore the raw sensations of pain and, as such, it is the vehicle through which you can begin to accept these messages. And when you do so, you will often find that pain waxes and wanes quite dramatically. There can be long moments of normality followed by flickers or spikes of pain. There are often different sensations too. Some are hot. Others cold. Some feel 'tight', others throb, while still others feel sharp or stabbing. Not all are completely unpleasant. The different sensations often rise and fall like the waves on the sea. They constantly change in character and intensity. By exploring each of these different sensations, moment by moment, you come to accept that they are like black clouds in the sky: you can watch as the sensations arise, drift past and disappear again. Your mind is like the sky and individual thoughts, feelings, emotions and sensations are like different types of cloud. So in a sense, mindfulness teaches you to observe the weather without becoming embroiled in it. And no matter what happens, the sky – your mind – remains untouched by it.

It is important to realise that mindful acceptance is not resignation to your fate. It is not the acceptance of the unacceptable. It is simply the acceptance of the situation as it is, for now, at least. It is a period of allowing, of letting be, of non-resistance, so that you cease to struggle. And when this struggle ceases, a sense of peace takes its place. Secondary Suffering then progressively diminishes. Often as not, Primary Suffering will begin to do so too.

We can explain this to you in minute detail. We can cite numerous scientific trials that prove the point. We could even show you scans of your own brain as it 'builds' the sensations of pain from all of your thoughts, feelings and emotions – but only when you have experienced the power of mindfulness for yourself will you truly believe it.

This is why it is called a *practice*. Accepting pain can be difficult. It's just better than the alternative, which is to live in a state of perpetual suffering.

Countless participants on our Breathworks courses have discovered this for themselves. Claire was one. She found that when her neck began to hurt she was also assailed by fear, anger, stress, sorrow, hopelessness, despair and exhaustion. So not only did she feel the initial unpleasant sensations in her neck, but she was also swamped with yet more suffering. It was almost as if she was struck with an arrow, and when she reacted to it she was then hit by a second one. Now she had to bear the pain of two arrows – that from the second being caused by *resistance* to the first. It is an entirely natural response. In fact, in cases of acute, rather than chronic, pain, it might even be the best response because it's a powerful driving force to take yourself out of danger. When it comes to chronic pain and illness, however, it is often precisely the wrong solution because it simply compounds your suffering. And, of course, it can then seem as if you're pierced not by two arrows, but by many, many more.

Accepting the sensations of Primary Suffering
allows the Secondary Suffering to take care of itself –
and to progressively diminish.

Claire discovered that she could resist pain for days or even weeks. She could distract herself with alcohol, cigarettes and food. She could squash the pain with powerful drugs. If those failed, she could ignore the pain – for a while, at least. But all this came at a cost: the rest of her life. She discovered that in ignoring and walling off the pain she had also isolated herself from all that is wonderful and precious about life. The world became increasingly wan and grey. Food lost its flavour and texture. She no longer laughed or cried. Her love life declined into irrelevance. All this meant that when she could no longer maintain the struggle, she simply crashed and burned. So not only did the pain return, but, with all of the things that normally sustained her love of life having evaporated, she was left feeling fragile and broken. No wonder her doctor wanted to prescribe her antidepressants.

After three years of struggling, Claire embraced mindfulness – not because she believed that it would work, but because she was desperate. And when she began to mindfully explore the sensations of pain, something remarkable and counter-intuitive began to happen. Not only did the pain begin to subside, but she began to experience all of the good things that had been squeezed out of her life too. It opened the door to a wealth of emotions such as happiness, love, compassion and empathy, as well as sadness. Claire realised that life is bittersweet, and when she let go of expecting it to be either wholly wonderful or truly distressing and to hold in an honest heart a delicate mixture of the two, she felt increasingly relaxed and open. Through facing up to and becoming sensitive to her own predicament, she became a happier and more centred person with greater empathy for others. She also began to heal.

OUR STORIES

Both of us have used mindfulness to help us cope with the pain, suffering and stress of serious accidents.

Vidyamala Burch's story

I had just turned twenty-three when I visited my parents' home in Wellington, New Zealand, for the Christmas holidays. Early on the morning of New Year's Day I was woken by the sound of a friend tapping at my window. He was driving to Auckland, where I lived, and offered me a lift. Still hung over from the previous night's celebrations, I slipped out quietly, leaving a note for my family, and fell asleep in the passenger seat.

The next thing I remembered was being trapped inside a mangled car, Tim's bloodied face beside me. He had fallen asleep at the wheel and we'd hit a telegraph pole. My shoulder was hurting, my neck was hurting, my arm was hurting ... and my back was hurting terribly. As well as the pain, I remember the sounds in the car. In the background, behind Tim's wailing, was another noise: the sound of my own screaming.

When I reached hospital I was told that I had a crushed collarbone, whiplash, concussion and other injuries. In time, these would prove to be the least of my worries, however, because I had also aggravated a serious spinal injury that I'd suffered six years previously and that had required two major operations. It would be another two years before X-rays revealed that the car accident had also fractured the middle of my spine. Whatever chance I might have had to live without chronic pain had been destroyed.

Pain, sometimes very intense, would become a central feature of my life for many years to come.

A few months after the accident, I returned to work as a film editor, but my whole spinal column was painful and I found working a physical and emotional strain. After two years of daily struggle, I reached a state of exhaustion and collapsed. The years of pushing and overriding my body had taken their toll. For months I didn't have the strength to even get out of bed. To make matters worse, I ended up in the intensive-care ward with serious complications, including a paralysed bladder. This was the scariest time of my life and the whole experience forced me to stop and take stock of everything.

The most intense time came during one long night in the hospital. I felt impaled on the edge of madness and it seemed that two voices were speaking within me. One was saying: *'I can't bear this. I'll go mad. There's no way I can endure this until morning.'* The other replied: *'You have to bear it; you have no choice.'* They argued incessantly, like a vice growing tighter every second. Then suddenly, out of the chaos came something new. I felt a powerful clarity and a third voice said: *'You don't have to get through until morning. You only have to get through the present moment.'*

This realisation transformed my experience. Tension opened into expansiveness as I understood the truth of what the third voice was saying. I knew, not intellectually, but in the marrow of my bones, that life can unfold only one moment at a time; I saw that the present moment is manageable, and I felt the confidence this knowledge brought. Fear drained out of me and I relaxed.

The next day the hospital chaplain – a man of deep kindness – visited me. He sat by my bed, held my hand and guided me through a visualisation in which he asked me to remember a time when I'd been happy. I took my mind back to holidays in New Zealand's South Island as a carefree teenager in love with the beauty of the high mountains. Through this, I made the profound discovery that, although my body was injured, my mind was still whole and I could experience peace. It was my first taste of the kind of calm mental clarity that accompanies mindfulness.

I realised that much of my torment had grown out of fear of the future – the future moments of pain that I imagined stretching on for ever – rather than what I was actually experiencing in the present moment. I was 'pre-feeling' my future pain and worry, as well as having to cope with present-moment suffering. I was needlessly multiplying my pain. Without understanding what had happened, I knew something extraordinary had broken through. It was a visceral experience that echoed through my thoughts and feelings – and it tasted of freedom.

I left hospital with a deep longing to investigate how I could use the mind to reduce my suffering. I started meditating regularly and gradually my life turned around and I became much happier. This meant I coped much better when things deteriorated further in 1997, when I became partially paraplegic with my bowel also becoming paralysed, and I had to start using crutches and a wheelchair to get around. A couple of years later I needed another big operation to rebuild my lower spine. This time I was much calmer. And when I saw the surgeon after a couple of years he was astonished at how well the new metalwork was holding up. This was because mindfulness had helped me to take care of my body – and my new metal spine – rather than abuse it, as I'd done previously.

When I thought back to how I'd struggled in my lowest times,

I knew that I wanted to reach out and help others who were coping with serious accidents and illnesses. So I decided to develop a mindfulness programme based on everything I'd learned. One of my main teachers was Dr Jon Kabat-Zinn, developer of Mindfulness-Based Stress Reduction (MBSR) and founder of the Stress Reduction Clinic at the University of Massachusetts Medical Center. Jon taught me an immense amount and encouraged my dream of establishing the Breathworks organisation to teach mindfulness to those suffering chronic pain and illness.

At Breathworks we developed the Mindfulness-Based Pain Management (MBPM) programme. Although originally designed to help people cope with the after-effects of accidents and illness, it also works extremely well for such mental pain as stress, anxiety and depression. MBPM is now available in many centres in over fifteen countries around the world including the UK, across Europe and Australasia. Breathworks has now become an international organisation that teaches and researches the uses of mindfulness in managing pain, illness and their accompanying stress.

When I look back at the girl I was in 1977 when I first injured my spine, it's as if a miracle has occurred. I now have a rich and fulfilling life in spite of my disability. I still have to take painkillers, though at a much lower dose than in my pre-mindfulness days, and I still have to use crutches and a wheelchair to get around (mindfulness obviously cannot repair a shattered spine). But I am at peace with my situation. I have a wonderful life that is largely free of secondary suffering. Mindfulness has given me these priceless gifts, and by writing this book with Danny I hope to share these techniques with you.

Danny Penman's story

My ordeal began when I was paragliding over the Cotswold hills in southern England. An unexpected gust of wind caught me off guard and collapsed the wing of my paraglider. One moment I was flying normally, the next I was tumbling head over heels into the hillside 30 feet below. I remember thinking with great calmness and clarity: '*Well, this probably isn't going to kill me, but it will hurt.*'

When I hit the hillside the world stopped turning. I felt cocooned in soft cotton wool. I opened my eyes and began to methodically check my body for damage. I made sure there was no sticky yellow fluid coming out of my ears or eyes (which would indicate a fractured skull) and that I could wiggle my fingers and toes. When I reached my legs I was struck with the most agonising pain imaginable. I soon realised why: the lower half of my right leg had been driven up through my knee and into my thigh. I could even see the outline of my fractured shin bone lifting the cloth of my jeans. I quickly went into shock and my body was wracked with violent uncontrollable spasms.

As I lay on the hillside, I remembered a form of meditation that I'd been taught in high school as a way of tackling exam nerves. Over the years I'd used it off and on to deal with the usual stresses and strains of daily life, but never in times of real physical pain and suffering. I knew that meditation had been used for pain relief, and as I lay on the hillside, in sheer desperation, I decided to give it a try.

I began by forcing myself to breathe slowly and deeply, to focus on the sensations the breath made as it flowed into and out of my body. I pictured myself in a beautiful garden, and imagined myself inhaling its peaceful and tranquil air as I did so. Gradually, breath by breath, the pain became more distant. It felt less 'personal', almost as if I was watching it on TV or through a thin mist, rather than experiencing it directly.

When I arrived in hospital it became apparent just how seriously injured I was – and just how effective a painkiller the meditation had been. The tibial plateau, or lower-knee joint, had broken into six pieces and the tibia and fibula (lower-leg bones) had shattered into six main fragments and numerous smaller chips. There was also significant damage to the muscles, tendons, ligaments and cartilage.

It turned out that I would need three major operations to rebuild my leg. I also needed a newly invented device, a Taylor Spatial Frame, to be surgically attached to my leg for six to eighteen months to repair the damage. Consisting of four equally spaced rings that encircled my lower leg, the frame looked like a cross between a Meccano set and a medieval torture device. Fourteen metal spokes and two bolts connected these rings to the shards of bone inside my leg. The spokes and rings of the frame could all move independently and allowed the surgeons to move bone fragments around inside my leg. In essence, the Taylor Spatial Frame replaced traditional hospital 'traction' and the plates and screws normally used to fix severely broken bones.

Life with the frame was intolerable. Sleep was virtually impossible and the pain from my injuries was controlled only with powerful drugs that left me washed out and jaded. I felt thoroughly wretched (not to mention anxious, irritable and highly stressed). It was clear that no amount of 'positive thinking' could shift such a traumatised state of mind, so I decided to find an alternative way of coping with the pain and of maximising my chances of recovery.

Because of my earlier experiences, I latched on to meditation as a possible treatment. I soon discovered the work of Mark Williams, Professor of Clinical Psychology at Oxford University in the UK. He and his co-workers at the Universities of Cambridge, Toronto and Massachusetts had spent over twenty years studying the phenomenal power of meditation for treating anxiety, stress, pain, exhaustion and even full-blown depression. They had turned it into a powerful therapy, known as Mindfulness-Based Cognitive Therapy.

I decided to try mindfulness meditation to help me cope with the after-effects of my accident. The simple meditation programme worked to an astonishing degree. My pain gradually subsided and I slashed my intake of painkillers by two-thirds. I also developed a more contented outlook on life, seeing my injuries as temporary problems that would gradually subside, rather than ones that might leave me confined to crutches or a wheelchair.

I'm convinced that mindfulness is the main reason why I recovered in double-quick time: the Taylor Spatial Frame was removed after just seventeen weeks (as opposed to the normal six to eighteen months). Certainly, my progress astonished my doctors. Shortly after my final operation I joked with the surgeon Mark Jackson, consultant at Bristol Royal Infirmary, that maybe my injuries hadn't been as bad as I'd thought. He looked at me aghast and said: 'Your leg was in the "top five" leg injuries I've treated with a Taylor Spatial Frame – and possibly higher.'

In 2008, at the age of forty-two, I took up running and hiked Britain's 630-mile South West Coast Path. I have no way of knowing how long such good fortune will last. My injuries still ache from time to time, but they no longer consume my life or prevent me from living it to the full. Mindfulness is not a panacea: it is simply a powerful therapy that dissolves pain and suffering. It allows your body to heal itself and helps you cope with the anxiety, stress and depression that so often accompany a serious illness or injury. I now accept each day as it comes and carry out the simple mental and physical exercises in the Breathworks programme.

CHAPTER THREE

Introducing the Mindfulness Programme

The final eight chapters of this book are dedicated to the mindfulness programme. Each of these chapters corresponds to one week of the programme. Each step will progressively soothe your suffering and settle your mind. Many people find that their pain begins to dissipate almost from the first week of the programme, although sometimes it can take a little longer. Any stress, anxiety or depression that you feel will also gradually dissolve, leaving you feeling re-energised and whole once again.

Each chapter contains two main elements. Firstly, there is the meditation programme itself, which takes twenty minutes per day. (You will find the meditation tracks on the CD that came with this book.) Detailed instructions for each of these practices are in the shaded boxes found in each chapter. This will allow you to read through the whole book and then to return to the meditation programme itself on a week-by-week basis. If you do read through the whole book, it is still best to reread each chapter before you start the corresponding week of the programme. Each week of the programme is built upon centuries of wisdom and some of the lessons can be subtle, so it is best if they are fresh in your mind.

The second element of the programme is the daily Habit Releasers. These progressively break down your negative habits of thinking and behaving. Habits can lock in place a substantial amount of pain, suffering and stress, so dissolving them enhances the effectiveness of the whole mindfulness programme. Habit Releasers are generally enjoyable to carry out and are designed to re-ignite your innate happiness and curiosity, while also melting away Secondary Suffering. Typical Habit Releasers consist of going to the park and soaking up the elements or waiting for the kettle to fully boil before making a cup of tea or coffee (rather than rushing to switch it off). Try to do these with your full attention – with full mindful awareness.

It is best to carry out the meditations on six days out of seven. It does not matter which days of the week you choose. If you miss out a day or two, simply try to make up the time on other days. You can then continue with the next week of the programme. If you should manage to meditate on only four days or fewer, then you should try to repeat that week of the programme if you can. Mindfulness gains its power through repetition, so it is important to meditate for the recommended number of days. However, life can be busy, so do not criticise yourself if you 'fail' to complete any part of the programme. You cannot 'fail' at meditation, but it can sometimes take a little longer to complete the whole programme than you might wish. If you should stall partway through the programme, again, try not to criticise yourself. Simply pick up the reins when you feel able. If many weeks or months have passed, then it's best to start again at week one.

And, if this should happen, try to remember that you have not failed. It is perfectly normal to pause, or to make repeated 'false' starts, on any mindfulness programme. A great many of those who are considered to have 'mastered' mindfulness initially did this. Paradoxical as it may seem, 'failing' and 'dropping out' can be important lessons in their own right. Compassion, particularly to yourself and the difficulties that you face, is a central feature of mindfulness. So try to avoid attacking yourself if you feel that you are not trying hard enough.

A week-by-week summary of the programme

Week One introduces the Body Scan meditation. As the name suggests, the meditation invites you to move your awareness around the body and to focus your mind on the sensations that you find. This simple meditation highlights the difference between *thinking* about a sensation and *experiencing* it directly. It helps you sense the difference between Primary and Secondary Suffering; your relationship with pain and illness will then change profoundly. For this reason, the Body Scan lays the foundations for the rest of the programme. This meditation is also an extremely powerful stress reliever.

Week Two introduces the simple Breathing Anchor meditation. This will help you become ever more aware of your thoughts, feelings and emotions as they arise in your mind – and to let go of struggling with them. You will learn that many of your thoughts and much of your behaviour are driven by the 'autopilot'. Most of your suffering is actually a habitual reaction to mental and physical 'triggers'. You can't get rid of these triggers but you can change how you react to them. The Breathing Anchor meditation helps you to do this. It will progressively teach you how to let go of your suffering so that you can begin living life to the full once again. This skill alone can change your life. Focusing on the breath in this way has other benefits too: it slowly dissolves anxiety, stress and depression and boosts physical healing by stimulating the parasympathetic or 'calming' aspect of the nervous system.

Week Three introduces the Mindful Movement meditation. Pain and illness have a significant impact on overall fitness, flexibility and the ability to carry out the ordinary tasks of daily life. While this is understandable, human bodies are designed to move, so if you don't remain as active as possible then you can begin suffering from a range of secondary health problems. Week Three introduces some very gentle mindful movement exercises that have been specially designed for the Breathworks programme. Broadly based on yoga and Pilates, they will forestall and even reverse the process of inactivity and help rebuild your confidence and courage. The emphasis throughout is on the *quality* of awareness as you carry out the movements, rather than aiming to bolster physical fitness (although they will do this as well). Week Three also encourages you to bring a measure of mindfulness, kindness and understanding towards your body as you go about your normal day-to-day activities. Once again, this will help you sense the difference between Primary and Secondary Suffering and further reduce your pain.

Week Four encourages you to turn towards your difficulties, rather than trying to avoid them. In most areas of everyday life, we tend to avoid or ignore the thoughts, feelings, emotions and sensations that we find difficult or unsettling. Week Four asks you to take a different approach with the Compassionate Acceptance meditation. This encourages you to gently face your difficulties and accept the things that you cannot change (Primary Suffering) and to reduce or overcome those that you can (Secondary Suffering). This acceptance is a period of allowing. Of letting be. Of bringing tenderness towards your 'failings' and difficulties. You will be surprised by the pain relief to be gained from simply bringing an attitude of warmth, compassion and gentle understanding towards yourself and the problems that you face.

Week Five gives you the tools to seek out the pleasant experiences that are so often masked by suffering. The previous week will have re-awakened your senses and allowed you to begin re-experiencing the world in all of its bittersweet beauty. Week Five builds on this skill with the Treasure of Pleasure meditation. Focusing your full awareness on such simple pleasures as the warmth of your hands or the taste of your favourite food can be transformative. Reducing pain and suffering is important, but it is equally vital that you begin to love life again.

Week Six builds on the previous two weeks with the Open Heart meditation. This will cultivate a confident, kind-hearted and broad awareness that dissipates pain and suffering. This enhanced sense of perspective will help you live in greater harmony with the world, rather than reacting to it and forever feeling on the back foot. This has profound implications for the management of your pain. It helps you to cease struggling against yourself, and the reality of your pain, suffering and stress, as you learn to be more compassionate towards yourself. And when you do so, a sense of peace and tranquillity fills the space. This is the cornerstone of Mindfulness-Based Pain Management.

Week Seven builds on the previous week by expanding your enhanced sense of kindness and compassion outwards from yourself to include other people. You might ask 'Why?' given that it is you who are suffering. It is simply because you *are* interconnected with other people whether you recognise it or not. We are social creatures. If we feel isolated then this enhances pain, suffering and stress, but the Connection meditation dissolves the sense of isolation that so often accompanies these experiences. It helps you to begin living in peace with yourself and others – no matter how physically isolated you are or feel yourself to be.

Week Eight marks the beginning of the rest of your life. It reviews the whole course and helps you build a mindfulness programme that is sustainable for the long term. It gently reminds you that although you can't control what happens in your life, you can choose how you respond.

A TIME AND A PLACE FOR MEDITATION

The meditations in this programme take only ten minutes and should, ideally, be carried out twice daily. It is up to you when you do them, but it is generally best to slot them in at the beginning and end of each day. Most people find early morning is best, shortly after getting up. Other good times are immediately after returning from work, or before the evening meal. This may mean that you have to rise a little earlier in the morning and, if you should do so, go to bed a little earlier too, so that the practice isn't carried out at the expense of sleep. Only you know your own natural cycles of alertness, sleepiness and suffering, so we'll leave it up to you to decide the best times. Regularity is important too. It cuts down on procrastination and allows you to schedule your day more efficiently. As the course progresses, you may also like to make your sessions a little longer – perhaps doing two meditations in a row in the morning or evening. But make sure you keep practising at least ten minutes at both ends of the day to maintain regularity.

If you feel overwhelmed, frantic or rushed, it is worth remembering that you probably do not have any spare time to meditate. If you did, the chances are you would already have allocated it to something else. You will therefore have to *make* time for it. Most people find that meditation tends to free up more time than it consumes because they live their life in a much smoother way and spend far less time suffering. Some people fear that meditation is 'self-indulgent' – that perhaps they should be spending the time with their family or working harder. In this sense, it is best to see your time meditating as being of benefit to both you *and* your family or friends. It is not self-indulgent or a waste. Quite the opposite. It will help you heal and regain control over your life and suffering, and is simply the most sensible and practical way of dealing with your pain, illness or stress. Another way of looking at mindfulness is to see it as mental exercise. Many people spend a lot of time exercising their body, but almost never try to maintain a measure of 'mind fitness'. Meditation is a fitness programme for the mind.

It is best to meditate in a pleasant and peaceful space. This can be as simple as a tranquil corner of your home. Sitting down amid mess and clutter won't help you develop inner clarity, whereas a clean and tidy space will help you cultivate a more contemplative state of mind. You may want to arrange a few flowers or ornaments in this area; or perhaps some pictures or an evocative natural object such as a rock or a piece of driftwood. It will also be helpful to turn off the telephone, switch it to silent, or divert it to voicemail, if that's appropriate. Finally, let others in your home know that you would like to remain undisturbed during your short periods of practice. Many people find this a little embarrassing, fearing that others will find mindfulness a little odd. In practice, your friends and family will be pleased that you are finding relief from your suffering and regaining control over your life.

And what will you need in the way of equipment? A CD or MP3 player to listen to the meditation tracks, a quiet space at home, a chair to sit on, or a rug to lie upon and possibly a blanket to place over your legs and feet to keep any chill at bay. This is all that you will need.

Some people find that they prefer to meditate in a group. If this is the case for you, you might like to join a local Breathworks course or follow one online (for an international list of accredited Breathworks trainers and course details visit www.breathworks-mindfulness.org.uk).

HOW SHOULD I SIT?

The word 'meditation' often brings to mind a picture of a supple young man or woman sitting cross-legged on the floor. While some people do meditate like this, it is frequently extremely uncomfortable. Sitting in such a position has nothing to do with the practice of meditation. It is simply the way people have traditionally sat in the East. As a consequence, it is best to carry out most of the meditations in this book while sitting on a straight-backed chair. If you find this difficult or uncomfortable, you can adopt one of the other positions detailed below. Try to accept your current physical situation and adapt to your own circumstances. You may find that lying down is best. Or you might like to try kneeling or sitting cross-legged. Choose a way that causes as little muscular strain as possible and encourages an alert but relaxed state of mind. Experiment until you find a posture conducive to meditation. Always try to remember to treat yourself with as much kindness and understanding as you can muster. Mindfulness is not a competition. You will gain nothing by forcing yourself into a harsh or uncomfortable position.

You may need to change your chosen posture as the weeks and months pass. This is not unusual. You may also need to shift positions part-way through a meditation. Again, this is not uncommon, especially if you have physical constraints. Even experienced meditators need to move from time to time. If you do move, try to include that in your meditation, moving as mindfully as you can.

Here are some ideas for choosing a meditation posture. Some of the descriptions might seem overly detailed. This is deliberate. If you meditate solely for stress relief, or to enhance mental health and wellbeing, then your overall posture is less critical. However, most people with chronic physical health problems have constraints that must be gingerly worked around, if only temporarily. This will ensure that you get as much benefit as possible from meditation, rather than spending your time struggling against discomfort. You can also access videos going over the principles of posture at www.breathworks-mindfulness.org.uk or www.franticworld.com

Sitting on a chair

Choose a chair that has a straight back. A wooden dining chair is ideal. If your spine is reasonably strong, try to sit an inch or two forward from the back of the chair. This will leave your spine free to follow its natural curves and create a sense of openness in the chest. It will also encourage alertness and emotional 'brightness'. If your back is weaker, you can place some cushions behind your spine to provide some support. Try to maintain as upright a posture as you can comfortably manage. Your feet should be flat on the floor. If your legs don't quite reach the ground, place a cushion or pillow under your feet so that they make firm and stable contact with the floor (below).

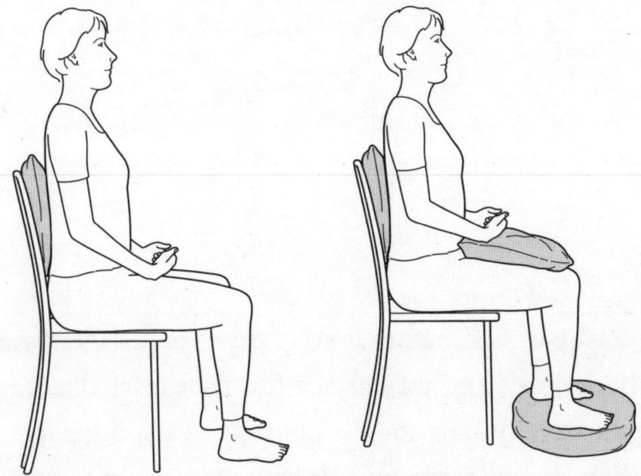

Balancing the pelvis

Whatever sitting posture you choose – in a chair, kneeling on the floor or sitting cross-legged – the key to finding a comfortable posture is the angle of your pelvis. The pelvis anchors the whole upper body and its angle affects the alignment of your head, neck and spine (see illustration overleaf). If you can find a posture in which the pelvis is balanced and erect, then the spine will follow its natural 'S' curve. This allows the head to rest lightly at the top of the spine and the back of the neck to be long and relaxed, with the chin slightly tucked in. A sense of openness will then arise quite naturally. A balanced pelvis also allows the legs to 'fall outwards' towards the floor and creates the least possible strain in the larger muscles of the thighs and hips.

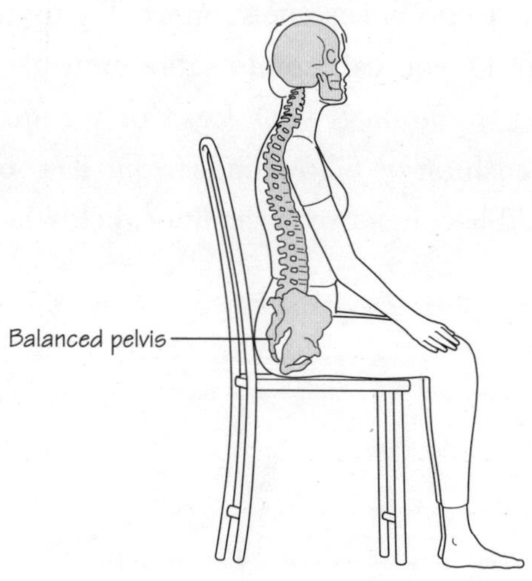

A good way of finding out if your pelvis is sufficiently erect is to tip it backwards and forwards a few times (see illustrations a and b opposite), looking for the point of rest and balance in the middle. You can also try putting your hands under the fleshy cheeks of the buttocks while seated and feeling for the sitting bones – the bony tips deep within the buttocks that take the weight as the body sits upright. When the pelvis is balanced, most of the weight passes directly through these bones, rather than via the fleshy pads at the back of the buttocks or the pubic area in front. Finding such a balanced posture can mean adjusting the height of your seat.

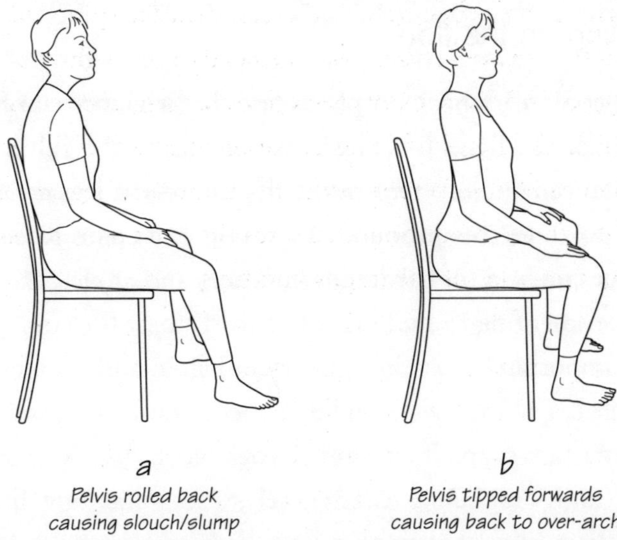

a Pelvis rolled back causing slouch/slump

b Pelvis tipped forwards causing back to over-arch

It's also important to rest your hands at the right height. You may want to support them on a cushion or have a blanket wrapped around you to help the shoulders remain open and broad instead of being drawn downwards as the meditation progresses (see illustrations c and d below).

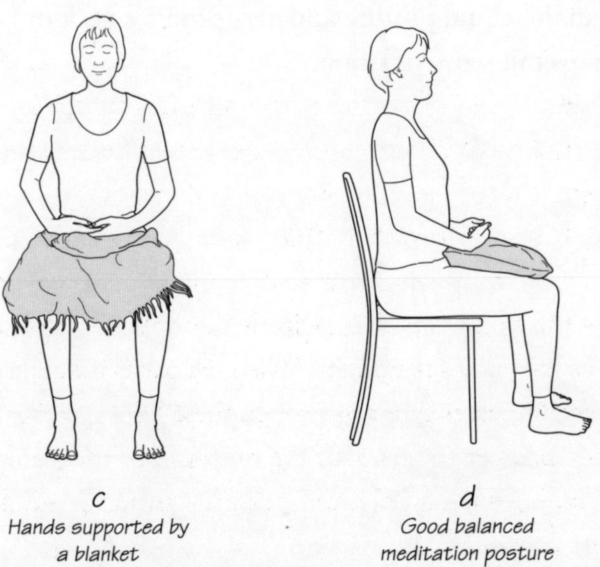

c Hands supported by a blanket

d Good balanced meditation posture

Kneeling on the floor

Some people with back problems find that it's more comfortable to kneel on the floor. It is often easier to adjust the pelvis so that it is balanced and erect when the thighs are at a less acute angle than the 90 degrees produced by sitting in a chair. Kneeling on the floor can be a bit harder on the knees and ankles, though, so try experimenting to find out what works best for you.

It is important to establish the right height and firmness while you kneel. You may want to buy a meditation stool, some meditation cushions, an air cushion or yoga blocks (see Resources for details and suppliers). Alternatively, use something firm and stable, such as a large book with a cushion on top for padding (see illustration e below). Your 'seat' should be neither too soft – which will make it unstable – nor too hard as this will be uncomfortable. If it's too high, your pelvis will tend to tip forwards, over-arching the lower back, and if it's too low, your pelvis may roll backwards, rounding the back and shoulders. Both extremes create an unhelpful posture and may produce neck or back pain and an overall sense of strain.

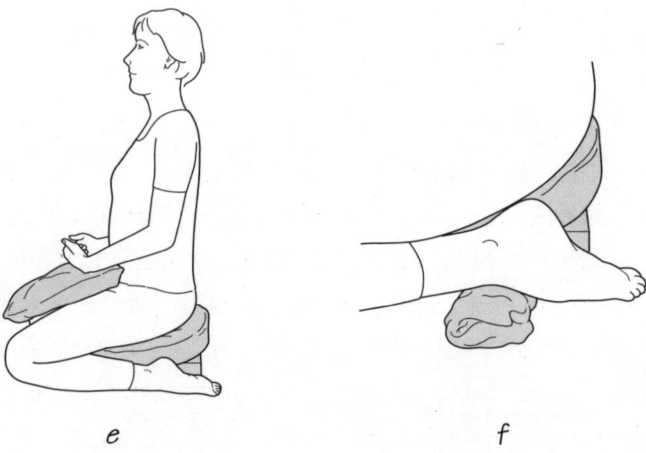

If you experience strain in your ankles while kneeling, try taking the strain off the joints by supporting them with rolled-up socks or something similar. Play around with what you have to hand and see what is most comfortable (see illustration f opposite).

Sitting cross-legged

By all means sit on the floor cross-legged if you find this comfortable. Apply all the same principles as for the other postures. Make sure your pelvis is balanced so your spine can follow its natural curves without either slouching or over-arching. Have your arms supported by either a cushion or blanket to minimise strain on the shoulders and neck (as in illustration e opposite).

In practice, sitting cross-legged requires a great deal of flexibility and is to be encouraged only if you can sit comfortably in this position without straining your body. It is often unsuitable for those dealing with chronic pain or health problems. So unless you're very flexible, sitting on a chair and kneeling on the floor are usually the two most desirable sitting meditation postures.

Lying down

The body scan meditation is generally carried out lying down, but this position is also best for other meditations if you find sitting on a chair uncomfortable. Lying on a mat on the floor is ideal. Sometimes it's best to avoid a bed as you will subconsciously associate it with sleep and may naturally become quite dozy. But if your bed is the only place you can be comfortable, then by all means meditate there.

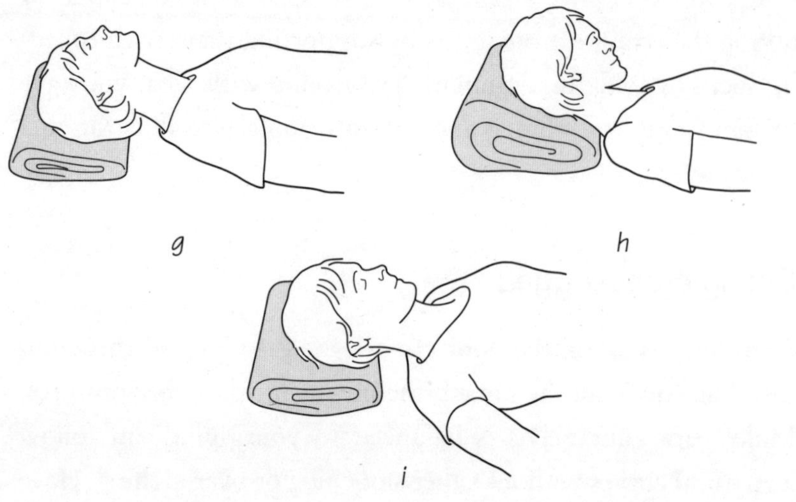

Make sure your head is at a comfortable height with the neck in a neutral position: use a firm cushion or folded blanket for support. And experiment to find a height that's neither too low, overstretching the front of the neck (see illustration g above), nor too high, overstretching the back of the neck (illustration h above). The optimum position (i) is where the forehead is slightly higher than the chin, allowing freedom in the neck by maintaining its natural curve.

To ease any strain on your back, raise the knees so the feet are flat on the floor (illustration j opposite). Alternatively, place a bolster, rolled blanket or cushions under the lower thighs and knees (k). Otherwise, lie with your legs outstretched (l).

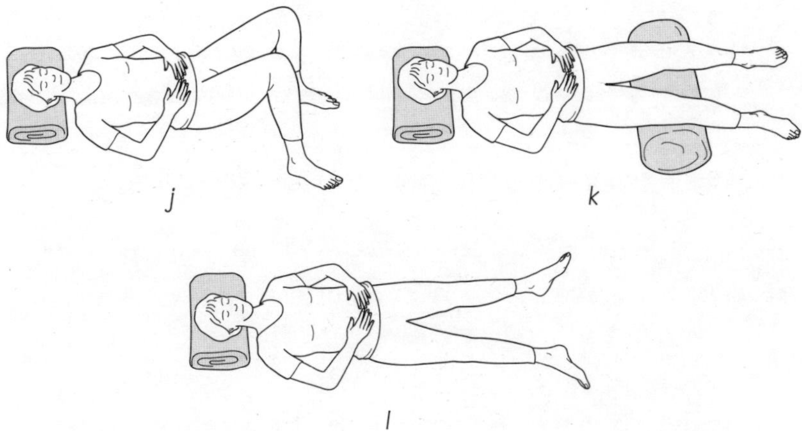

WHEN WILL YOU BEGIN THE PROGRAMME?

If you are wondering when to start your practice, why not begin now? After all, the present moment is the future that you promised yourself last year, last week, yesterday ... Now is the only moment that you will ever have.

If you can't start this moment, why not do the Coffee meditation below during your next break and then decide when you will begin?

The Coffee meditation

Coffee and tea are drinks that we take for granted, which makes them ideal subjects for meditation. You can use this meditation to settle the mind before making a decision or simply to gain a glimpse of mindful awareness. Repeat it whenever you choose or do it with any drink at all.

- If you are making the drink yourself, look closely at the coffee grounds (or tea leaves). Really observe them. Spend a few moments letting your eyes soak up every detail. Observe how the light bounces off the grounds or leaves.
- Add the water. What can you hear? What can you smell? If you are buying your drink, soak up all of the sounds and smells of the café. Can you hear tinkling cups? The hiss of water? The chatter of other customers? Try to tune directly into your senses, rather than mentally describing the experience in words.
- If you are adding milk and sugar, watch how they dissolve. Does the smell change? Focus on the subtly different aromas.
- Take a sip. Coffee has over thirty different flavours and tea has many more. See if you can sense some of them. Are there some bitter notes, sweet ones, sour ones ... ?
- Resist the temptation to gulp down that sip; instead, after a few moments, or when you feel that your taste buds have become saturated, swallow it. How does it feel? When you breathe in, how do your mouth and throat feel? Hot? Cold? Or hot followed by cold?
- Repeat the previous two steps with another sip of your drink. Carry on repeating this for five minutes or until you've finished your drink.

How do you feel? Is it different from normal? Did the drink taste better than if you had consumed it at your normal speed?

CHAPTER FOUR

Week One: Wild Horses

'Misery was just normal for years after it happened,' says Mike. 'I was a welder in a shipyard. It's not like in the old days when it was hard graft in the open air. These days it's a high-tech operation carried out in covered dry docks. The steel is cut by laser and there are sophisticated gantries to hold it in place while it's welded. That was the problem. I'd become so unfit and stiff over the years that I was an injury waiting to happen.'

Mike was welding a piece of sheet steel on to a freighter when he turned to look over his shoulder. He felt a sharp tug in his lower back. Although it hurt, he thought nothing more of it until he went for a cup of tea an hour later. By then, his whole lower back had stiffened up. A few hours later he was in agony every time he moved. Even breathing was painful. It was the start of a five-year ordeal which saw him being referred from specialist to specialist and from pain clinic to pain clinic.

Before his accident, Mike had become increasingly divorced from his body. It had become little more than a vehicle for carrying his brain around. This was hardly surprising. His job – and life in general – had all seduced him into forgetting his body and its needs.

Mike's job was highly skilled and relied on his using specialised machines and equipment. His work was performed as much in his head as with his body. The range of movements his body was required to carry out had progressively shrunk over the years. He'd begun to fossilise, even though the mental tempo of his work had increased significantly. He became increasingly stressed and often felt like he was drowning. Mike had become a cog in an enormous machine.

It's easy to spend so much time inside your own head that you can forget you have a body. You spend so much time thinking that the outside world might as well not exist at all. Thinking, worrying, comparing and judging can consume so much of your time that you begin to lose a sense of the body. This is compounded by the 'always on' world of TV, radio, Internet, smartphones and social media that keeps us connected to the outside world – but not to our own inner one.

But there's a further problem too. You might have subconsciously begun to avoid your body. In your heart might lie a sense that you don't like yours so much. And this may be deepened by the beautiful (and airbrushed) images that bombard us from films, TV programmes and magazines. By comparison, your own body might not be as slim or as strong as you would like. It might not be as tall or as beautiful or handsome as you want. And day by day, you learn that it is not as young as it once was. So there might be a tendency in your heart to ignore your body as much as possible. This tendency is increased if you've spent years suffering with chronic pain. Chances are, you've turned your pain into a demon to be avoided at all costs. And there might also be a sense of fear: that one day your body might fail catastrophically. Most of us dare not admit that one day we will die.

Such a disconnect between mind and body might not appear to matter so much, but it masks a critical problem: it means that you have lost a vital skill. It means that you are no longer capable of 'calibrating' the different feelings that the mind builds into the sensations of pleasure, pain and suffering. So when you suffer an accident – or a serious illness – it's almost as if a rusty valve is opened in the brain's pain centres that can't be closed again. Your sensations can start to behave like one of those faulty old showers that alternate between bursts of scalding-hot and ice-cold water. This, more than anything else, is the driving force behind the Secondary Suffering that we discussed in Chapter Two. And it makes the pain that you actually feel infinitely worse.

Whether you like it or not, you do have a body, and if you ignore it, or deny it, then you are only storing up problems for yourself. It is not possible to ignore your body for ever. Eventually, it will demand attention, even if it is only through the natural aches and pains of ageing. For this reason, the first step of the Mindfulness programme is to gingerly make contact with the body again. As you do this, your suffering will gradually begin to subside. First to go, inch by inch, will be your mental torment and its accompanying stress. Then your Secondary Suffering will begin to dissolve. Finally, as you progress through the weeks ahead, you will experience a lessening of Primary Suffering; the raw physical sensations that the brain builds into the visceral sensations of pain.

At this stage, no one can say whether your pain will disappear completely. But almost everyone who practises mindfulness for health reasons experiences a significant lessening in their overall pain and distress. And virtually everyone feels reconnected with life again. Quite simply, life becomes worth living once more.

And this is what Mike learned: 'I thought it was normal to be miserable,' he says. 'The pain meant that I started to drink a lot and always had a hangover. So then I thought that it was normal to feel sick and have a headache as well. I didn't know that it was possible to enjoy life. I'd completely forgotten about that bit of being alive. This is what mindfulness gave me. Most of my pain went but, more importantly, I started to enjoy life again.'

Practices for Week One

- Ten minutes of the Body Scan meditation (see page 63; track 1 on the CD) to be carried out twice per day.
- A Habit Releaser: spend a little time with nature each day (see page 74).

THE BODY SCAN

The Body Scan begins the process of reintegrating your mind and body. This is crucial for distinguishing between Primary and Secondary Suffering, and, ultimately, reducing the pain that you actually suffer. It will also begin the process of dissolving stress along with any anxiety or depression that you are feeling.

The meditation invites you to gently move your awareness around your body, region by region, and to observe, with as much objectivity as you can, what you find. The idea is to hold each area centre stage for a while, before gently letting go and moving on to the next. It encourages you to bring, as best you can, a calm and inquisitive flavour of awareness to the meditation. Try to leave behind any preconceptions about what you 'should' feel and instead try to simply observe what you find. You might find areas that are numb. Other regions might be burning or throbbing. You might discover stabbing pains or perhaps a dull ache. It is not unusual to find areas of calm neutrality; a sense of pulsating life. Try to feel whether the sensations are fixed and unchanging or if they flux from moment to moment. You may be surprised to discover that your pain is not a 'solid' enemy, but is somehow more 'fluid' than that. If it's possible, try to get a sense of the thoughts and emotions that accompany these sensations. Fear, anger and sorrow are common. These might be accompanied by anxious, stressed and depressed thoughts. But relief and a sense of peace and happiness might also be found. Whatever you find, try not to judge it in any way. As best you can, simply observe. When you do this, you will notice your suffering and stress begin to gradually soften and dissolve. After a while, you will discover that:

Relaxation is your natural state
when you stop creating tension.

Try to be as kind and understanding towards yourself as you can. If you are slightly fearful or anxious about what you will find, remember that you don't have to jump into the meditation with both feet. Be an explorer. Move inch by inch, and only as far as you feel able. Meditation is neither a marathon nor a sprint, but should be seen as a gentle ramble that encourages you to move at your own pace.

Remember that if any sensations become too unpleasant you can move your body to relieve your suffering. Make a conscious choice about how you will respond. You can try changing position or relaxing into the pain. See if the ebb and flow of the breath affects the pain. Often the breath will help dissolve your suffering. Always try to remember that you are free to do whatever you require to be comfortable. The practice will be far more beneficial if you are relaxed, rather than fighting pain or discomfort.

As you progress through the meditation you will notice that it asks you to pay particular attention to the breath. This is a common theme that runs through the whole programme. The breath is not only the source of life, but is also a sensitive barometer for any emotions or physical sensations that you are feeling just below the threshold of awareness. With practice, you can learn to use the breath as an early-warning system that allows you to sense and defuse suffering and stress before they become a problem. Often, simply observing the breath – making sure it is as natural as possible – can dissolve pain, suffering and stress without your needing to do anything else at all.

To gain a sense of how powerful this effect can be, try the following: clench your fist and notice what happens to the breath. You'll probably find that you hold your breath and that it feels frozen in the abdomen. Now, relax around your breath and breathe into the sensations of clenching. Do you notice how your fist relaxes a little as well?

Most people automatically hold their breath when they feel pain, stress or discomfort. The habit of inhibiting the breath can also manifest as shallow breathing or as hyperventilation. Such disturbed breathing triggers the mind's alarm systems, which, in turn, create tension and stress in the body. The mind then senses this increase in tension and stress and becomes even more alarmed. In this way, disturbed breathing can drive Secondary Suffering in a vicious and distressing cycle that also fuels anxiety and stress. The reverse is also true: breathing into pain or distressing feelings tends to dissolve them. So mindfulness and breath awareness can be used to sap this vicious cycle of its momentum. Very quickly, your distress spins down into a state of peacefulness.

Mindfulness works on another deeper and more physiological level too. When you pay attention to the breath, and it becomes calmer, it naturally becomes deeper and more rhythmic. You also start to use the back of your lungs and ribcage a little more. In fact, your whole back moves when you breathe naturally. Combined with the movements in the chest and abdomen, along with the massaging of the internal organs with each breath, this is known as 'whole-body breathing'. This is naturally calming.[1] It stimulates the parasympathetic nervous system, which releases many hormones into the body that defuse tension and stress and promote healing. In turn, this creates deep-seated feelings of peacefulness and relaxation. These feelings then encourage more whole-body breathing. This virtuous cycle is also an extremely powerful antidote to pain, suffering, stress and anxiety.

Central to the whole-body breathing is awareness of the movement of the diaphragm, which rests deep within the body, lying beneath the lungs and across the body from side to side and front to back.

On the in-breath, the diaphragm broadens and flattens down inside the body, causing the lungs to fill with air. On the out-breath, the diaphragm relaxes, causing the lungs to empty and expel their stale air (see page 60).

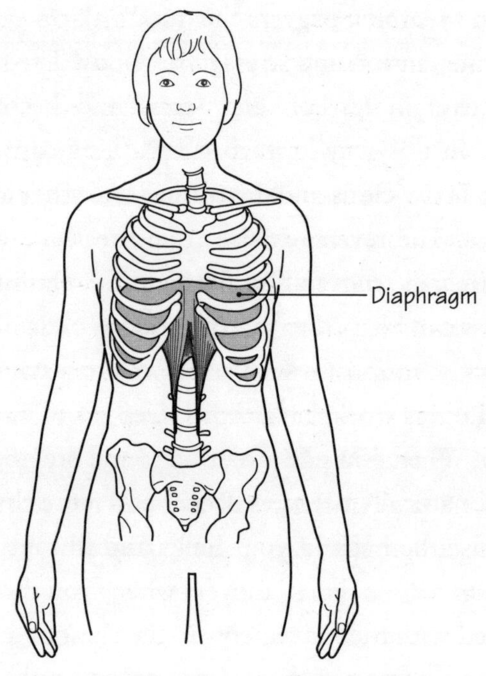

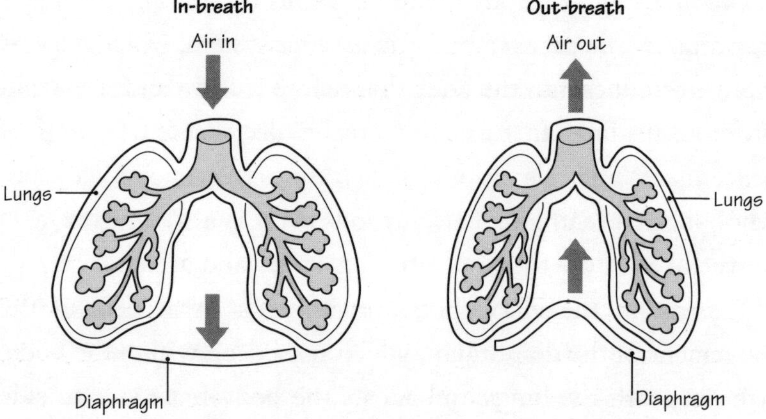

When you do the Body Scan, it encourages you to feel the breath and then to soften around it as you guide your awareness through the different parts of your body. You may notice that you quickly revert to inhibiting and tightening around the breath in areas that are tense or painful. You will have probably turned this tightening into quite a persistent habit. This is normal, so try not to criticise yourself. Instead, simply soften this tension with a gentle inward smile each time you notice it. Breathing into the experience of pain or distress – imaginatively directing your breathing towards the unpleasantness – naturally undermines the habit of inhibiting the breath. It is then a great relief to simply let go and relax into the out-breath. Gradually, during the course of a few breaths, your tension will begin to reduce. This is also true for emotional distress. Feeling stressed, anxious or depressed is often associated with a contracted breath. Calm and peacefulness naturally arise when you become aware of this tendency and then simply breathe into the emotional tension.

Gradually, you will learn to breathe more deeply and naturally. People often report that this ability to breathe anew changes their life more significantly than anything else.

If you want more detailed guidance on the physiology of breathing, please go to www.breathworks-mindfulness.org.uk or www.franticworld.com

Practicalities

The Body Scan meditation takes only ten minutes and should be performed twice per day on six days out of the next seven. The best times are in the morning and in the evening (or perhaps the afternoon). It is also preferable to carry them out at the same times each day. It is important to establish a routine, as this will support you on those days when your energy or enthusiasm is lacking. Most people find it useful to read through the meditation guidance on page 63 before actually doing it, and then carrying it out while listening to the CD (track 1). As your experience deepens you may like to try other versions of the Body Scan (these are available on www.breathworks-mindfulness.org.uk).

It is worth refreshing your mind about the practicalities of meditation (see pages 41–51). It is best carried out in warm and quiet surroundings, and remember to arrange to not be disturbed. For example, you might want to let others in your home know when you are meditating. You should also switch off your phone or set it to divert to voicemail.

It is perfectly normal when starting a mindfulness programme to feel resistance. Your mind may suddenly find many new and more pressing matters to attend to. You might start to feel guilty about devoting time to meditation. If this should happen, remind yourself that this is *your* time that has been set aside to heal and nourish *you*. And remember that when you begin to heal, everyone around you will benefit too. If resistance should still persist, then gently remind yourself of what others have found: *mindfulness tends to liberate more time than it consumes.*

It does this by breaking down many of the habits of thinking and behaving that consume so much of the day. These force you to run over the same ground over and over again. As you become more aware of the workings of your mind and body, you will start to notice how much of your life is run by the autopilot. And when you do so, you then have the option of stepping off the treadmill and using your time for other things. As you progress through the programme, you'll find that you are becoming more and more efficient at home and at work.

Body Scan meditation

This week you'll learn a Body Scan meditation that places particular emphasis on the sensations of breathing as you guide your awareness through the whole body.

Preparation

Adopt as comfortable a position as possible, perhaps covering yourself with a light blanket if this will help you feel more warm and relaxed.

Most people prefer to do the body scan lying down, but if this is uncomfortable for you, then by all means do it sitting in a chair or even standing. If you feel particular pain or discomfort during the meditation, feel free to adjust your position. The meditation instructions assume that you are lying down. If you are doing it in another position, then adapt as necessary.

Allow your body to settle down on to the bed or floor as much as you can. Place your arms at the sides of your body with your hands very gently resting on your belly.

Allow your shoulders to rest back towards the floor with your face soft and the eyes lightly closed, if this is comfortable, and your hands soft.

Have your legs outstretched, or if you've got a lower-back problem you may prefer to put some pillows or cushions behind each knee to take the strain off the area, or you can bend the knees with the feet flat on the floor, hip width apart in the semi-supine position. Do whatever is most comfortable for you.

As you begin to settle, can you give your weight fully up to gravity, allowing it to gently draw your body down towards the floor and the earth?

The scan

Begin by tuning into the movement of the breath beneath the hands. Can you feel your belly swelling a little on the in-breath and subsiding a little on the out-breath? Be careful not to alter or force the breath, but rest your awareness within its natural movements. And what about the chest? Can you feel the ribs expanding on the in-breath and retracting on the out-breath? Can you get a sense of the lungs filling and emptying within the chest with each breath?

Between the chest and the abdomen there's a large muscle called the diaphragm that rests across the body from side to side and front to back. On the in-breath the diaphragm broadens and flattens down inside the body; and on the out-breath it relaxes back up to rest beneath the lungs again, shaped a little like an umbrella or a parachute. The diaphragm moves ceaselessly from the moment of birth to the moment of death and, as it broadens and flattens within the body on the in-breath, it gently pushes down on the internal organs, causing the belly to swell outwards. And as the diaphragm relaxes back up inside the body on the out-breath, the internal organs subside back into the body again and the belly does so too. Can you get a sense of this movement beneath your hands as they rest on your belly? Try to follow the movement without forcing the breath in any way.

And can you get any sense of an echo of the breath down in the pelvic floor? This is the diamond-shaped area between the anus at the back, the urinary organs at the front and the buttocks on either side. The echo of the breath will be very subtle, so don't worry if you can't feel anything at all. But over time, you may become receptive to a very subtle broadening and opening on the in-breath and retracting and toning on the out-breath, with the whole pelvic-floor area a little soft and relaxed. This won't be a physical or muscular movement. It's utterly receptive, more of the nature of an ocean swell.

Now allow your awareness to inhabit the buttocks. If you notice they're tense, then you might also notice how it's quite natural to relax and soften tension when you become aware of it, allowing the buttocks to be soft against the bed or the floor.

And allow your awareness to inhabit the lower back, the middle back and the upper back as they rest on the floor or bed, follow their natural curves and shape.

Now see if you can get any sense of the breath in the whole back of the body. As the diaphragm moves within the body it involves the back of the body as well as the front. Be curious about what you can feel in your back with the breath. What do you notice? Maybe you can even feel the echo of the breath in the lower back. If you've got any pain or discomfort in your lower back, can you allow it to be massaged by the breath, a breath that is saturated with gentleness and kindliness – bathing the lower back in tenderness? Respond to your own discomfort as you would naturally respond to a loved one who was hurting.

And can you feel the movement of the ribs in the back of the body? Expanding on the in-breath and retracting on the out-breath. Perhaps reflect for a moment on how the ribs and the lungs are as much in the back of the body as the front. Maybe this is a new idea for you – but becoming aware of the movement of the breath in the back of the body is naturally calming; can you get a sense of this?

Now allow your awareness to inhabit your shoulders as they drop back towards the bed or floor so they're fully supported. And can you allow the arms to gently fall away from the shoulders? Allow your awareness to inhabit the upper arms, the elbows, the lower arms and the hands. And allow your awareness to flow inside the fingers and thumbs, resting your awareness there for a few moments.

Now coming back up the arms, allow your awareness to flow into the throat and back of the neck and the sides of the neck. Allow your awareness to inhabit the whole head and face. Can you let your head be heavy, fully supported by the cushion or pillow it's resting on?

And what do you notice in your face? If you notice tension, do you find it natural to soften and release it in the light of awareness? Soft lips, soft tongue, soft cheeks, soft eyes.

Can you allow the back of the mouth and the top of the throat to be soft, letting the breath flow freely in and out? Can you let your jaw hang a little loosely, unclenching the teeth? This may help this area feel a bit softer and more receptive to the flow of the breath.

And now, guiding your awareness down through the body to the hips, allow the legs to gently fall away from the hips. Let the legs be fully supported by the bed or floor, whether you've got your legs outstretched or you're lying in a semi-supine position. Giving the weight of your legs up to gravity, allow awareness to flow into the front, back and sides of the thighs.

And now allow awareness to flow down to inhabit the knees . . . and the lower legs . . . the ankles . . . the soles of the feet . . . the tops of the feet. Can you invite your awareness right inside your toes? What do you feel there? Maybe it feels intense or maybe it feels dull or numb. It doesn't matter. What matters is that you are aware.

And now broaden out your awareness to inhabit the whole body. The legs . . . the torso – front, back and sides . . . the arms, the neck and the head.

Can you get a sense of the breath in the whole body? Very gently expanding on the in-breath and subsiding on the out-breath. If you've got pain or discomfort, can you let these areas be gently massaged and soothed by the gentle rhythm of the natural breath – allowing the breath to be saturated with tenderness and kindliness?

As you rest within the natural and continual flow of movement in the body with the natural breath, you may notice how sensations are also continually changing. What you think of as 'pain' or 'discomfort' is actually changing sensations coming into being and passing away, moment by moment, and you only ever experience this flow of sensations one moment at a time. 'Pain' or 'discomfort' is not as solid as we often think. Can you get a sense of how sensations are fluid, like the breath, as you rest within the breathing body, resting within a sense of change and flow in your whole body, moment by moment, as you allow the breath to be gentle, tender and kindly.

Conclusion

And now gradually bring this short breath-based Body Scan to a close. Open your eyes and gently and carefully move your body. Perhaps form an intention to take this more fluid and pliable awareness of your body with you as you gradually re-engage with the activities of your day. Allow your experience to be saturated with a kindly, gentle breath, no matter what you're engaged in.

FRANTIC THOUGHTS

Did you find that the Body Scan helped your mind settle and become calm like a still pool? Or did you discover that thoughts rampaged across your mind like a wild bull? Virtually everyone's mind wanders while meditating. This is entirely normal. It's what minds do. Steffen had to remind himself of this repeatedly: 'I remembered the meditation teacher telling us that mindfulness is not about success or failure. Becoming aware of your wandering mind is a sign that mindfulness is beginning to take root. It's a lesson I had to learn for myself again and again and again.'

As Steffen discovered, the moment that you become aware that your mind has wandered is a moment of mindfulness. It's a sign that you're moving away from the autopilot towards a more considered state of mind – one that allows you to see the world more clearly and helps you to respond more effectively. With practice, these 'magic moments' of full consciousness become more frequent and join together in a flow of awareness. This helps to dissolve suffering by gently soothing the brain's pain networks. As these pain circuits calm down, you also become more aware of your life as it happens, rather than always being stuck in the past or fantasising about the future. And this, in turn, tends to damp down feelings of 'drowning' under a tide of stress and anxiety.

When your mind wanders in this way, try as best you can to shepherd your awareness back to the body and the breath. Try to be as understanding as possible. Your mind *will* repeatedly wander. And there is nothing to be gained from punishing it for doing what it is designed to do; instead, try to work *with* your mind. Try inviting it back to the body or breath with a sense of curiosity. Encourage it to discover what can be found in the continuous flow of life through your body. A good way of visualising this approach is to contrast the two ways that wild horses are trained in America's Midwest.

Patience and the wild mustang

One approach to taming a wild mustang is to break its spirit. It can be beaten into submission by yoking it to a post and then violently yanking on its bit and bridle until the animal is bent to the trainer's will. This does work, in a way, but the horse becomes sullen and suspicious.

A gentler approach is that epitomised by Monty Roberts – a 'horse whisperer' who trains wild animals by becoming attuned to their language. He tamed a wild mustang colt on the great plains of America.[2] The mustang was strong, and if Monty had used force he'd have become embroiled in an impossible battle. Instead, he allowed the colt to run and run while he followed behind on his own horse. He let the mustang go wherever it wished. The colt eventually slowed and acknowledged his presence. At that point, Monty stopped his pursuit and went in the opposite direction. The wild horse then began to follow out of curiosity. Within two days, Monty had earned the horse's trust and just hours later a rider was on its back.

If your mind behaves with the free spirit of a mustang, try to adopt a similar approach to Monty's. If you try to force your mind to become still, it will kick and buck wildly. You will become exhausted by the struggle. If, however, you let the mind roam, and follow it with your awareness, it will settle down of its own accord. Your mind struggles only because you oppose it. If you are patient, and focus your awareness on the mind's struggle, then it will become calm. You can then refocus your awareness on the breath – or body – and the mind will start to become curious about the object of your meditation. It will behave just like the wild mustang that's been naturally tamed – gentle and calm, yet alert and vibrant.

There may also be another reason why your mind refuses to settle, especially if your body is in pain or highly stressed while you do the meditation. It is entirely natural for the mind to avoid unpleasant sensations in the body. It will continuously try to distract your attention. In fact, it will probably do all in its power to *not* pay attention to the unpleasant sensations. In technical parlance, this is known as aversion. When you begin to pay attention to the unpleasant sensations, and your mind begins to behave like a wild mustang, begin to observe the way that your mind works. Pay attention to your thoughts and the way that they hop from subject to subject. Watch how it drags up troubling memories and extrapolates them into the future, creating anxiety, stress and sadness along the way. For a short while, simply observe the developing patterns. Try giving them names such as 'thinking, thinking', 'worrying, worrying' or 'painful thoughts, painful thoughts'. After you've watched your thoughts for a short while, gently coax your mind back to the breath and continue with the meditation.

OTHER EXPERIENCES YOU MAY ENCOUNTER

Sometimes the Body Scan can initially make you feel worse, not better. This is also a good sign. A good way of looking at it is to see your pain as an enormous bag of shopping that you have been carrying around without rest. When you put the shopping down, what is the first thing that you feel? There is a sense of relief, but often there is quite a bit of pain too as your hands uncurl and stretch. This is because all of your muscles, tendons and ligaments begin to relax and unfurl of their own accord, resuming their natural alignments once again. So for a while, your suffering actually increases. This is what can happen with the Body Scan. As you relax, your body has to adjust to a lack of tension and stress. If you have spent years suffering with pain, tension and stress, then it can take a while for your body to return to its natural healthy balance of shape and alignment. After a while, when your body has resumed its natural alignments, your pain will begin to reduce – often quite substantially.

Going to sleep

Jess found that she felt tired after meditating. Claire frequently fell asleep part-way through. These are not 'problems', but are actually signs of heightened awareness. It means that your mind and body are reconnecting. If you have spent years suffering, then it is natural to feel exhausted. It is only when stress begins to dissolve that this exhaustion bubbles to the surface. If this is the case, don't criticise yourself in any way. Congratulate yourself on having caught up on a little sleep and continue the meditation where you left off. If you feel tired after the meditation, try to accept the situation and go to bed a little earlier. Over time, you will start to notice a renewed sense of energy in your life. You can also use this sleepiness to your advantage if you suffer from insomnia. Simply use the body scan when you go to bed to get a better night's sleep.

Feeling panicky

Toby had the opposite problem. He would occasionally feel fear, or even panic: 'I wasn't used to being quiet and still. It was very unpleasant, but it soon passed.' Toby learned that by slowing his out-breaths and relaxing the weight of his body into the floor he could gain a sense of 'grounding'. This reassured him that he was safe in the room. He also mentally reminded himself that such feelings soon pass.

Awareness of the breath in daily life

Once an hour, stop and be still for a few moments. Take your awareness inside your body to rest on the physical sensations of the breath. If you notice that you're holding your breath, see if you can relax it a little. You can also bring awareness to the breath as you go about everyday life. Each time you notice that you're holding your breath against pain or discomfort, practise breathing into these sensations with gentleness and tenderness, softening the breath and relaxing any tension that you feel.

When Mike did this, he realised something simple, but profound. He noticed that the breath is always changing and this was something that his mind found increasingly interesting. He became fascinated by how breathing is felt as a constant flow of movement and sensations. He was able to relate this to his pain and discomfort. These too changed continuously – never exactly the same from one moment to the next. In this way he changed his relationship to his pain: rather than seeing it as a static enemy to be defeated, he softened around it and experienced it as a process of changing sensations.

'Lots of people tense up when they feel their pain', says Mike. 'They're afraid of it and try to avoid it. But you shouldn't be afraid, if you can help it. It takes some guts to look at your pain, but when you do, you realise that it's not hard or solid or unchanging. It's like the breath – and everything else in life – it changes moment by moment. Often it's not as bad as you think it's going to be. When I looked more closely, the pain began to dissolve. Sometimes, it was pleasant in an unexpected way. I found warmth, tingling and a form of muscle tightness that felt like I'd just taken some healthy exercise.'

The act of simply watching your pain with calm acceptance can begin to transform suffering. It does this by helping you to relate differently to painful sensations. As we saw in Chapter Two, you can begin to see them as akin to changing weather patterns in the sky. Sometimes there is a violent storm. Other times there are clouds on an otherwise sunny day. But one thing remains constant: the sky. The weather may change, but the sky always remains. Mike began to see his mind as the sky and his pain as the weather. Pain, like the weather, is ever changing. And sometimes, there is not a cloud in the sky.

HABIT RELEASER: SPEND A LITTLE TIME WITH NATURE

The natural world is a powerful stress reliever and mood booster. It puts things in perspective and soothes even the most frayed of nerves. For these reasons, this week's Habit Releaser is to spend a little time each day with nature while being aware of the different feelings and sensations of the breath in your body. You can spend your time in a local park or nature reserve or, if you are feeling a little more adventurous, go somewhere wilder such as the mountains or the seashore. The important thing is to soak up the natural surroundings as mindfully as you can. If you are housebound, then look out of the window and soak up the view in exactly the same way or perhaps imagine being out in nature.

When you arrive at your chosen location, spend a few minutes absorbing the scene. What can you see, hear and smell? Does the air have a taste? How do the earth, grass and tree bark feel? Are they rough, smooth, soft or slippery? When you feel safe, on a park bench perhaps, close your eyes and focus on the sounds. Soak up the different ones. Can you hear the wind? Or perhaps the notes of different car engines in the distance? Can you hear insects, birdsong or the scampering of small animals such as squirrels? Notice the rise and fall of each individual sound. Mentally flick between them.

Can you feel the weight of your body settling on to the park bench or whatever you're sitting on? Can you give your weight up to gravity so that you feel a sense of rest? Can you feel the movement of the breath in your whole body – the front, the back and the sides? Can you feel how the breath is always changing, just as the sounds do? Can you let any sensations of discomfort in the body also come and go as the moments pass? See if you can have a more fluid experience of both your body and the world around you.

If you are physically able, take a short walk. Feel the sensations underfoot and notice the movement of your muscles and joints. Feel the gentle swaying of your limbs. Remember, though, the aim is to walk mindfully, not to push yourself physically.

Do this Habit Releaser every day this week, or at least six days out of seven. Spend as much time as you wish each time you do so, but it's best to be with nature for at least ten minutes. If you find that you can't manage to go each day, then try to go at least once this week and spend a whole hour, if you are up to it. Nature will reward you well.

CHAPTER FIVE

Week Two: You Are Not Your Thoughts

Just outside Vancouver on Canada's west coast stands the Capilano Canyon suspension bridge. It's 70 metres high, extremely narrow and sways to an alarming degree in the wind. In 1974 two researchers, Donald Dutton and Arthur Aron, placed a young and pretty student in the centre of the bridge. Her job was to ask male passers-by to complete a questionnaire. At the end of each survey, the young woman handed over her home telephone number to the man concerned and said that she would happily discuss the study in further detail with him that evening. This being a psychology experiment, there was more to the survey than met the eye. It was, in fact, an investigation into how our interpretation of bodily sensations such as a racing heart can affect what we think, feel and even how we behave.

It turned out that half of the Capilano men telephoned the

young woman that evening, while only one-eighth of those who were asked on a more stable bridge made the call. This was because the men on the Capilano bridge had mistaken their sweaty palms, elevated heart rate and trembling knees for sexual attraction – fear was confused with desire. In technical parlance, this is known as the 'misattribution of arousal'. And it turns out that many of our physical sensations and emotions can be misattributed in such a manner.

Dutton and Aron's experiments reveal something curious about our inner lives: we do not simply experience a physical sensation as if it were a free-standing and objective 'thing', but we also attach our own 'meaning' to it so that it becomes part of our emotional landscape. It even influences the thoughts that flow across our mind. This is because thoughts, physical sensations and emotions are all intimately connected. They feed back on each other – often in surprising ways and in quite distressing directions. For example, studies show that feelings of anxiety, stress, depression and exhaustion can create physical pain, make us more sensitive to it and make it far more unpleasant than it need be. These findings are of more than just academic interest because they also offer you a way out of your suffering. For if you can ease your stress and emotional pain using mindfulness, then you can also significantly reduce your physical suffering too. Here's how.

VICIOUS EMOTIONAL CYCLES

Experiencing an emotion is a multi-step process. Take fear as an example. When we sense a threat, the heart rate increases and the body tenses up readying us to either fight, run away or freeze. This is the unconscious 'fight, flight or freeze' response – and it works in quite a curious way. In fact, the decision to fight, flee or freeze is taken as much by the body as the brain. For example, if the body senses danger then the heart rate increases and the whole body becomes primed for action. The mind then senses the body's reaction – a racing heart while crossing a swaying bridge, for example – and triggers an emotional response. We then consciously recognise the emotion, and often as not, give it a label such as fear, anger, worry, love, etc. The process is so fast and seamless that these steps seem to be one and the same. So in practice, it is the emotion that we become aware of, while all of the body's reactions continue bubbling away in the background. We tend to notice the fear, love or anger, rather than the underlying rush of hormones and elevated blood pressure. This seems straightforward until you realise that we sometimes misinterpret our body's sensations and give them the wrong label, as the Capilano bridge experiment demonstrated.

Virtually all of the time, the mind makes the correct interpretation – unless, that is, you've spent years suffering with chronic pain, illness or stress. Take the example of pain. In this case your brain has become fine-tuned to spot the first flickerings of pain. You're on the lookout for the first hint of pain so that you can take steps to avoid the worst of it. In practice this means that when your brain spots something that looks like pain, it turns up its sensory amplifiers to the maximum for a closer look and also primes the body for action. This stress reaction then makes the body tense up, aggravating any aches, pains, illnesses and injuries. This, in turn, makes the body even more sensitive to pain. It triggers a vicious cycle. It's Secondary Suffering gone wild.

To make matters even worse, these responses can become hard-wired into your brain so that you end up seeing everything through a 'pain-tinted' lens. It becomes ever easier to feel pain and, when you do feel it, it is far more intense than it needs to be. So it becomes ever harder to become pain-free. In a sense, your brain has learned to automate your suffering. It has turned into a habit. You can see this effect in a brain scanner. People who've spent years suffering have more nervous tissue in their brain's pain matrix. This is the part of the brain that produces the conscious sensations of pain. Their brain's pain matrix has adapted in the same way as a muscle adapts to exercise – it's grown bigger and stronger. It's almost as if the years of suffering have made their 'pain muscles' grow in size so that they are more efficient at suffering.

This is not to say that pain is somehow your fault, that it is a figment of your imagination or that you are 'making it up'. Nothing could be further from the truth. Your pain is absolutely real. We are not trying to negate or 'explain away' your suffering. We are explaining how the mind perceives pain, so that you can understand how mindfulness unties the knots that hold your suffering in place. And once you understand this, you are on the road to eliminating much of your pain, suffering and stress.

When you're suffering, it's not just emotions and physical sensations that are interconnected: the conscious mind can get involved too. When you are in pain, it is quite natural to seek a way out. When you do so, you deploy one of your mind's most powerful tools – rational critical thinking. It works like this. You see yourself in a place (in pain) and you know where you want to be (healthy and pain-free). Your mind then analyses the gap between the two and tries to bridge it. This fires up the mind's

Doing mode (psychologists call it this because it performs well in solving problems and getting things done).[1] The Doing mode works by progressively closing the gap between where you are and where you want to be. It does this by breaking down the problem into small pieces, then analysing and solving them, before finally reassessing the problem to see whether the solution has got you closer to your goal.

The Doing mode often works in an instant, before you are even aware of it. It's a fantastically powerful process that helps you solve countless different types of problems, from navigating across a city to arranging a hectic work schedule. In a more refined form it's how engineers design ever more fuel-efficient cars and how doctors treat disease.

The Doing mode is without doubt one of humanity's most important assets, so it is entirely natural to apply this approach to finding relief from pain. However, when it comes to chronic pain and suffering, using the mind's Doing mode is the worst thing you can do. This is because by forcing you to focus on the gap between where you are and where you want to be, it is highlighting that gap. And if the gap can't be closed because you've already tried everything that medicine has to offer, you can end up in a mental cul-de-sac. You become increasingly fixated on the gap and unable to find an escape – you are trapped like a rabbit in a car's headlights – and can end up torturing yourself with harsh critical questions that grind away at your soul: '*Why does it hurt so much?*'; '*What's started it this time?*'; '*Is it getting even worse?*'; '*It hurts – what have I done to myself this time?*'

Such open-ended questions can enhance anxiety, stress and depression. They burn up your energy, leaving you feeling fragile and broken. But it's often worse than this because such questions also give the mind free rein to explain its darkest fears.

You can end up thinking: *'It'll get worse and worse ... I don't know what's going on ... Nobody knows what's going on ... My life will be ruined. Maybe I'll never get better ... Maybe its terminal and they haven't noticed ... Maybe they just won't give me the bad news ...'*

One fear leads to the next, which leads to the next and then the next. Before you know it, you can become lost inside a maze of dark and maudlin thoughts. But such a vicious cycle isn't just a terrible mental and emotional experience – it's also a crippling one. Mental torment amplifies physical pain and suffering. And physical pain and suffering feed back again to increase your mental anguish. It's an endless cycle that can leave you burned out and exhausted.

But there is an alternative ...

If you have a chronic health condition, or suffer from stress, you cannot stop the triggering of unpleasant sensations in the body. But you can stop what happens next. You can stop the spiral of negative thoughts, feelings and emotions that drive your pain. It is possible to relate differently to your suffering. And when you do so, you'll find that your suffering begins to evaporate. You can do this by harnessing an alternative to the mind's Doing mode. We rely so much on the Doing mode that we often forget that we are also *aware*. We are so used to relating to the world by filtering it through our thoughts that we forget about the magical property of consciousness. You can become *aware* that you are thinking. Scientists call this *metacognition* and it allows you to experience the world directly without your thoughts acting as a lens. It's like a vantage point that allows you to see your mind in action. Or a mountaintop that's unclouded by thoughts, feelings and emotions. Psychologists call it the Being mode of mind.[2]

The Being mode allows you to step back from your pain and suffering. It helps you break free of the tendency to *over-think* about your pain and suffering. It stops your thoughts acting as a filter or a distorting lens and breaks the cycle that leads to anxiety, stress, depression – and, ultimately, more pain.

Being mode is not better or worse than the Doing mode, just different. It's bigger than thinking. Kinder than thinking. And can often be wiser than thinking too. For thousands of years, people have learned to cultivate this Being mode, and it is possible for any of us to do the same through the practice of mindfulness meditation.

Mindful awareness – or mindfulness – arises out of this Being mode when we learn to pay kindly attention, on purpose, in the present moment, without harsh judgement, to things as they actually are.

Through mindfulness you can learn to see the world – and your suffering – as it *actually* is, not as you expect it to be or fear it might become. And when you do so, something quite remarkable will happen: your pain will begin to diminish and might even go completely. Even if some of your suffering should remain, research shows that it will bother you far, far less.[3]

At this stage, some of these ideas might be a little too nebulous to grasp. If this is the case, don't worry – the Being mode and the ideas it embodies can often become a little rusty through under-use. These ideas will, however, become a little clearer as you progress through the programme. 'Belief' is irrelevant. Simply carry out the practices and your pain and suffering will begin to dissolve.

Main Characteristics of the Doing and Being Modes

1. **Automatic pilot versus conscious choice:** the Doing mode is brilliant at automating your life by creating habits. Such habits are extremely useful for carrying out repetitive tasks such as washing the dishes or driving, because they free up 'mindspace' for other tasks. The trouble is, they can begin to automate your entire life, so that you start to live in your head, rather than the real world. It can automate what you think, feel and sense. It can also automate how you behave and relate to others and the world in general. Your whole life can become one long series of interlinked habits with very little conscious input. Even suffering can become a habit. The Being mode brings you back to full conscious awareness. It puts you back in contact with all of your senses. You directly sense the world around you, instead of simply thinking about it. This awareness tends to dissolve habits, so that you can begin to consciously live life to the full again.

2. **Analysing versus sensing:** the Doing mode analyses the world. It thinks, plans, remembers, compares and judges. These are all vital skills, but they can backfire if taken to extremes. You can begin to live inside your own thoughts and lose contact with the world. Such 'over-thinking' can go tragically wrong and enhance mental and physical suffering. It's one of the root causes of anxiety, stress, depression and exhaustion. These forms of mental anguish can add further to pain and suffering in an endless vicious cycle. Mindfulness – the Being mode – is a truly different way of knowing the world. It puts you back in

contact with your senses so that you gain an intuitive knowledge of the world. It helps you to 'live in the moment', rather than being trapped in the past or worrying about the future. It soothes your tired and 'over-thinking' mind so that it can begin to rejuvenate itself.

3. **Avoidance versus approaching:** the Doing mode works by holding on to your goals, but also by bearing in mind 'anti-goals' – the things that you want to avoid. This is an extremely powerful way of solving problems. If navigating across a city, for example, it's useful to know which areas to avoid. When it comes to chronic pain, suffering and stress, however, it can make matters worse. By trying to avoid such difficulties you can compound them by adding an extra layer of fears, worries and insecurities. You can start to fixate on them so that they begin to consume the mind. This is the heart of Secondary Suffering.

   Being mode dissolves fears and worries by giving you the courage and space to approach them. It invites you to bring a compassionate curiosity to your most difficult states of mind and body. It does not say 'Don't worry' or 'Don't feel pain', but instead encourages you to bring a warm-hearted awareness to these difficulties. Often, your darkest fears never come to pass and simply evaporate when you embrace them with a calm and compassionate mind.

4. **Striving versus accepting:** the Doing mode compares the world with a version that exists only in your hopes, dreams, fears and nightmares. It focuses on the gap between the two and tries to bridge it. The Being mode accepts the world as it

is. This is not a form of resignation, but a simple acceptance – or assessment – of the situation as it is right now. It leads to a calmer and healthier state of mind and body.

5. **Viewing thoughts as 'solid' and 'real' versus viewing them as 'mental events':** the Doing mode uses thoughts and ideas as its currency. One thought builds on the next and the next. It creates ideas about the world and tests them in the mind's eye. This is, again, a tremendously powerful way of solving problems, but your mind can mistake these ideas for reality. Mindfulness teaches us that thoughts are just thoughts. They are just passing mental events. They might accurately reflect the world and your suffering – but they might not. Thinking is often important and thoughts are valuable, but not always. Thoughts are not 'you' or 'reality'. Thoughts are not necessarily true – even the ones that claim to be. Another way of describing this is learning to look 'at' your thoughts, rather than 'from' them.

Restoring balance

Doing and Being modes of mind are equally important but have different roles to play. In the West we have traditionally focused on using the Doing mode so much that it has become over-developed. It's a bit like a bodybuilder who has focused all of his efforts in building up the strength of one leg and neglected the other. Very soon all he can do is run around in circles – very quickly. Mindfulness helps to restore balance.

BECOMING A HUMAN BEING

In Chapter Four, the first week of the mindfulness programme began the process of re-integrating your mind and body. You will have learned that the breath and bodily sensations are in constant flux. Pain, like every other sensation, is neither constant nor static but always changing, so you only ever need to experience it one moment at a time. This realisation can give you a first taste of the difference between Primary and Secondary Suffering. As this distinction sinks in, you will find that your suffering begins to decline. And anxiety, stress and depression will begin melting away too.

The next step is to take these ideas further and deeper. A key aspect of mindfulness is gaining a sense of perspective on your moment-to-moment experience. Just like physical sensations, thoughts and emotions are also in constant flux. This constant 'chatter' of thoughts is the mind's Doing mode in action. Becoming aware of this chatter as an 'outside' observer with a clear sense of perspective – rather than feeling part of the 'story' – is the mind's Being mode in action. It is the mind's chatter that tends to create suffering, while simply observing the chatter as it comes and goes, and being less identified with the precise content of the mind, gradually dissolves pain and stress. Observing this process as it unfolds before your mind's eye is a tremendously liberating experience. It will also lead to the realisation that pain is simply one aspect of your daily experience. Unpleasant? Yes. The totality of your life? No.

Becoming a human being not a human doing

Sheila told us about her transition from a 'human doing' to a 'human being':

> In the space of two years I've had a brain tumour, a spinal tumour, osteoporosis and degenerative lung disease, and went from working full-time in a busy job and having many hobbies to being mostly housebound and taking large doses of morphine to manage the pain. But the hardest thing is the immense fatigue the brain tumour causes.
>
> I've always been 'driven', moving at speed from one task to another. The jobs list I set for myself each day is fearsome and, I'm realising, completely unrealistic for somebody like me who's ill. I struggle through a few things on my list and get ever more frustrated at what I haven't achieved. I was expecting the Mindfulness for Health course just to help me with pain control, but it's changing my whole way of looking at life. I'm discovering that I need to develop other ways of living and to look at the qualities that make life worthwhile, not the number of tasks I complete.
>
> This week my tutor asked me to develop more spaciousness around activities. I'm learning that it's possible to feel loved and supported for who I *am*, not what I can *do*. I'm learning for the first time in my life that I am a human being and not a human doing!

Practices for Week Two

- Ten minutes of the Body Scan meditation (see page 63; track 1 on the CD), to be carried out on six days out of the next seven.
- Ten minutes of the Breathing Anchor meditation (see page 92; track 2 on the CD), to be carried out on six days out of the next seven. This should ideally be done at a different time of day to the Body Scan meditation. If you choose, you can also do an extra Body Scan immediately before the Breathing Anchor meditation to help settle your the mind and body.
- A Habit Releaser: watch the sky for a while (see page 100).

BREATHING ANCHOR

The Breathing Anchor meditation, which is introduced this week, reveals the mind's Doing mode in action. It allows you to observe the workings of your own mind, so that you can see how it creates needless suffering by tying itself in knots. The meditation teaches you to observe your thoughts – to look 'at' them instead of seeing the world from 'inside' them – so that you experience the world directly, rather than seeing it through a lens tinged with pain, stress and worry. This is the Being mode. And it frees you from the autopilot that has mechanised so much of your suffering. Many people say that it's one of the most important skills they gain from the whole programme.

How can focusing on the breath achieve such profound benefits?

- Firstly, it teaches you that you can relate to pain, illness and stress in the same way as you relate to the breath. You can take a breath only for this moment. It is impossible to take a breath for the past. Or for the future. Past and future breaths are just ideas, not experiences. As far as the breath is concerned, only this moment exists. And you can relate to pain and suffering in the same way. Pain need be experienced only one moment at a time. Suffering is different – you can amplify it with painful memories or project it into the future to make it even worse. You can carry it around with you almost as if it was a tank of oxygen ready to feed your pain. But focusing on the breath brings you back to the present moment and teaches you a subtly different way of relating to a commonplace experience. And, ultimately, it helps you learn to distinguish between Primary and Secondary Suffering.

- Secondly, it provides a dynamic anchor for your awareness. It allows you to see when your mind has wandered and the gentle movements of the breath in the body provide a focus to return to. This gradually builds your powers of mindful awareness – where the mind, body and heart are an integrated whole, rather than fragmented. This awareness will serve as the bedrock for the rest of the programme.

- Thirdly, the breath teaches us that we do not always need to be in control. The breath breathes itself. It matters very little who we are or what we want to achieve. You can simply relax and take life as it comes. Not needing to be in control – and therefore not fearing a loss of control – is a liberating experience in itself. Stress simply melts away in the face of this realisation. You will gradually learn to take this feeling of calm tranquillity with you wherever you go simply because the breath is always with you.

- Fourthly, you may also become aware of a nagging tendency to want to 'fix things'. By not rushing in to put things right, but just resting your awareness on the breath, you learn that a great many things do not need to be fixed immediately. Some things can be left alone to play out as they will. This is an important skill to learn in its own right.

- Fifthly, the breath can be a sensitive emotional radar, as we saw in Chapter Four (see page 58). When you are stressed, anxious or in pain, the breath can be held for quite long periods without your realising it, or it may alternate between being fast and shallow, or deep and laboured. All of our emotions are reflected in the breath, but we are often unaware of it. By focusing on the breath while paying attention to your own emotional landscape, you can learn to use these sensations as an early-warning system. It allows you to detect the first stirrings of Secondary Suffering. Simply dropping your awareness into the breath at regular points through the day can give you enough warning to head off anxiety, stress, depression and exhaustion.

Practicalities

This week there are two meditations to carry out. The first is the Body Scan (track 1). This is identical to the one you did last week. The second is the Breathing Anchor (track 2). Each takes ten minutes and should be carried out at least once per day and be done at different times from each other. For example, you might like to do the Breathing Anchor in the morning and the Body Scan in the evening. You can do the meditations whenever you choose, although it is preferable to carry them out at the same times each day.

It is also worth refreshing your mind about the practicalities of meditation (see pages 41–51): the practices are best carried out in warm and quiet surroundings, so if possible arrange not to be disturbed. You might want to let others in your home know when you are meditating. You should also switch off your phone or set it to divert to voicemail.

As with last week's meditation, it is best if you read through the meditation guidance before you carry it out. And when you come to actually do the meditation, it's best to do it while listening to the audio track. This week you might also like to extend your meditation experience by sitting or lying for a short while after the audio track has finished. Many people do this quite naturally. If you cannot do it, try not to criticise yourself or feel guilty in any way. It's an option, nothing more. Another option is to do an extra Body Scan immediately before the Breathing Anchor meditation to help you settle the mind and body. This will deepen your experience. If you have an MP3 player, you may want to create a playlist to make it easier. If you do this, make sure the combined meditation is just one of your daily sessions. You should still do another session at a different time of day. If you like, you can also access different versions of both the Body Scan and Breathing Anchor meditations (log on to www.breathworks-mindfulness.org.uk or www.franticworld.com).

Breathing Anchor meditation

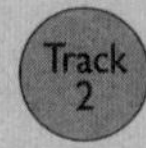

Adopt as comfortable a position as possible. It is often best to carry this out while sitting, but you can do it in any posture: standing, lying, sitting or even walking. Although the guidance will assume you are sitting, simply adapt the instructions as you go along to whatever posture you've chosen.

Sitting on a chair with your back upright yet relaxed, with your spine following its natural curves, see if you can establish a position that feels dignified, awake, alert and yet relaxed.

Allow your body to settle, to rest down into gravity, letting it be held and supported by the floor beneath you. And gently close your eyes, if that's comfortable. This will help your awareness settle and quieten by lessening external distractions.

The meditation

Gradually allow your awareness to gather around the sensations of the breath in your body. Where do you feel the breath most strongly? Be curious about your actual experience, letting go of what you think should be happening and being with your experience without judgement.

Now very gently rest your awareness within the whole torso. Can you feel your belly swelling a little on the in-breath and subsiding on the out-breath? Can you feel any movement and sensations with the breath in the sides and in the back of the body as well? Gradually inhabit your body a little more deeply with a sense of kindly curiosity towards whatever you're experiencing as you breathe. Remember to be accepting of whatever is happening. See if you can cultivate a precise awareness of the sensations and movement of the breath in the body as they happen, moment by moment, being careful not to force or strain. Allow your awareness to be utterly receptive as it rests upon the natural movement of the breath in the body. Allow the breath to be saturated with kindliness and tenderness as it rocks and cradles the body – soothing any stress, pain or discomfort you may feel.

Now become aware of any thoughts and emotions. Remember that meditation isn't about having a blank or empty mind. It's normal to think. Meditation is a training whereby you cultivate awareness of what is actually happening physically, mentally and emotionally, so you can gradually change your perspective and feel like you have more choice in how you relate to life. Can you look 'at' your thoughts and emotions rather than 'from' them? Can you get a sense of being aware of what you are thinking and feeling without either blocking your experience on the one hand or getting lost or overwhelmed by it on the other?

And don't forget that thoughts are not facts – even those that say they are. As you develop perspective on your thoughts and emotions, including repetitive undermining thoughts and feelings, can you let go of being so caught up in them? Notice how they're continually changing one moment to the next in exactly the same way as your breath is always changing. They're not as fixed and solid as you perhaps thought.

Using awareness of the movement and sensations of the breath in your body as an anchor for the mind over and over again, follow the breath all the way in and all the way out. And each time your awareness wanders, as it will, simply note this and return to the breathing anchor – time after time after time, moment by moment, making sure that you're very kind and patient with yourself. Even if you have to start again a hundred times, it's OK. This is what the training is all about. And remember that each time you notice that you've wandered, this is a magic moment of awareness: a moment where you've woken up from a distraction. A moment of choice. So when you catch yourself having wandered off, you're succeeding in the practice, not failing; just as you are succeeding when you manage to stay with the breath.

What's happening now? What are you thinking? Just note this and guide your awareness back to the sensation of the breath and the body, over and over again.

Conclusion

Gently begin to bring the meditation to a close. Open your eyes and be aware of the sounds around you – inside and outside the room. Feel your whole body and gradually, gently, begin to move, making sure you give yourself time to make a smooth transition from the meditation to whatever you're doing next.

ALIVE AND KICKING

After a few days of using the Breathing Anchor, Karen felt her body return to life again. 'I know it sounds stupid, but I thought to myself: *I am alive*. I felt fully connected to my body for the first time in years. There was something about becoming aware of the breath, experienced directly as sensations and movement in the body, that was relaxing and eye-opening at the same time. It was something I hadn't experienced before.'

Karen realised that no matter how worried or stressed she might feel, these states of mind are like the breath: always flowing. Anxiety, stress, depression, exhaustion and suffering all arise and then depart. At the time, they might seem like solid immovable facts – and persuasive ones at that – but not all thoughts are accurate, even those that claim to be. Even pain ebbs and flows.

Karen knew this on an intellectual level. She had read several books on meditation and understood the underlying concepts. She knew that thoughts are not facts and that 'you are not your thoughts'. Still, she didn't feel this enhanced sense of perspective in her bones. It was only when she persisted with the programme and began the Breathing Anchor meditation that the message was brought home to her. Karen learned that you can't experience a breath from the past nor one from the future. The only one you can really experience is *this* breath, happening right here in the body, right *now*.

'It was like an epiphany for me,' she says. 'I realised that I was projecting my current distress into the far future, so that I assumed I would be suffering for ever. I was totally preoccupied with how much I'd suffered in the past too. Meditation helped me to see that I could treat my suffering in the same way as the breath. I need not "pre-feel" my future pain or dwell on my previous bouts of suffering. All I have to do is get through this moment. When you realise this then most of your suffering seems to evaporate. It just goes.

'I also understood that much of my mental pain, my stress and depression, were the result of the disconnection between my mind and body. I simply could not relate to what was happening right *now* in the real world. I felt disconnected from life.'

This disconnection took the form of a harsh, driving voice

that constantly chided Karen. It criticised her for being weak. For giving in to the pain. It was her mind's Doing mode in action. Meditation offered her an alternative: the Being mode. It was a path between actively avoiding it and trying to squash it out of existence. This allowed her to gently explore her pain in a place of safety. She learned to breathe into the areas of tension with the aim of softening them. At first, it took a conscious effort to breathe into painful areas and not to be afraid. The first time she tried, Karen found herself gently crying with the release of emotional tension. But when she began to experience her pain directly, rather than mediated through distressing thoughts and emotions, she realised that it wasn't as widespread as she'd feared. Instead of feeling that the whole left side of her body and neck hurt, she saw that there were certain 'hot spots' of intensity. And even these were not painful all of the time. This was a revelation because she had always assumed it to be 'solid' and a fundamental part of her as a person. Equally surprising was the discovery that sometimes the pain felt 'loud' and sometimes 'soft'. Sometimes it was 'jagged' and at other times it was 'tingly' like pins and needles.

When Karen began to explore her own pain, she discovered something unexpected. She realised that she could breathe softly into it with tenderness. She approached it as a mother soothes her crying child. It was her first real experience of self-compassion. For the first time in her life she was able to say with a tender inner voice: *How have I got myself into this state of pain?* It was dramatically different from her usual inner critic, which was always barbed with criticism, barking: *You're really stupid getting so stressed about things. No one else gets into such a state.*

In a strange way, Karen's harsh inner critic was trying to help.

It was attempting to fortify her in the only way it knew how. So rather than confronting her critical inner voice, she embraced it instead. After all, this barking voice was part of her too. She calmly observed its torment, and little by little, this part of her simply settled down, withdrew its claws, and stopped gnashing its teeth. It was almost as if it knew that it was no longer needed as her protector.

After a while, Karen realised that the meditation was working on a more direct physical level too. It was not only dissolving the mental torment that led to Secondary Suffering, but was having a direct physiological benefit. It had actually begun to reduce her Primary Suffering too. When she focused on the movement of the breath, it started to flow more smoothly and began to gently massage her body's sore points. So rather than thinking, *It hurts, it hurts,* she began to think, *It's not the whole side of my body that's hurting, it's just some sore points. It's amazing my breath reaches so far. The body is amazing, there is so much happening all of the time.* She was astonished to discover that almost all of the body is connected to the breath in some way. The body moves continuously and the breath is its driving force.

THE BREATH REVEALS THE DOING MODE

While Karen was stressed and in pain she would withdraw from the world, but Jamie did the opposite – and he didn't realise it until he was halfway through Week Two. When his pain and stress began to build, he would start hitting out at those around him. He assumed that the world was in some way conspiring against him to heighten his stress and suffering. His anger was entirely understandable. Pain *is* unfair and *does* appear intolerable, so anger is a natural reaction. But it was also counter-productive because it quickly turned inwards and began to consume him.

When his smashed knees began to ache mercilessly, he blamed it on the weather, on 'useless bloody painkillers', on not being able to do his physiotherapy or just plain bad luck. Jamie's family knew that his anger was only making his pain worse, but it was a revelation to him.

His mental funk would always begin the same way. He'd start comparing himself with other people. Jamie would look at his co-workers – and even friends – with a highly critical eye. He'd imagine that their lives were perfect. He'd become increasingly annoyed that they earned more than he did, that they had 'better' houses and cars. But most of all, he hated the fact that their lives were pain-free, while his was a constant fog of aching and suffering. This turmoil aggravated the pain of his smashed 'rugby player's knees'.

He eventually realised that this was his mind's Doing mode in action. And when one day this clicked in his mind – at about the point in the programme where you are now – he simply stopped and breathed deeply. His stress began to fall away almost immediately. He remembered that it is impossible for the mind's Doing mode to operate while awareness is focused on moment-to-moment sensations. He understood that you can't be lost in thoughts and aware of the body in the same moment. And now, whenever he notices that his mind has begun to ruminate, he consciously drops his awareness back into the breath. As he breathes in, he says to himself, 'this breath' and when he breathes out he says, 'this moment'. It's a reminder for him to take stock of the world as it is, not through the lens of his turbulent negative thought patterns.

Experiencing the fluid nature of life

On one day this week, every hour, stop and be still for a few moments. See if you can be aware of the fluid and changing nature of sensations, thoughts and emotions. Feel the contact between your feet and the floor. Let your weight drop downwards as you surrender your body to gravity. When your mind wanders, as it surely will, bring your awareness back to the fluid and changing nature of your thoughts, sensations and emotions. See how they change as you go about your everyday life.

As well as stopping and breathing deeply, another technique Jamie learned is to consciously name the states of mind he is experiencing. 'I found it useful when my mind wandered during meditation to mentally say to myself, "thinking, thinking" or "fearful thoughts, fearful thoughts". I took this one stage further and began to do this when I noticed stress through the day.'

Objectively observing and naming thoughts and feelings as they arise helped Jamie to see that thoughts, feelings and painful sensations were not 'him' – but were simply one temporary aspect of his character. By observing his thoughts, he found that he could separate himself from them. It was he who was doing the observing and naming, rather than the one being named. Instead of saying, 'I'm stressed', he came to realise that he was feeling some of the symptoms of stress. He learned that his life was not defined by pain and suffering, but that he sometimes – often even – experienced pain and suffering. This may seem like a distinction without a difference, but it had huge practical consequences. It allowed Jamie to put a thin sliver of space between him and whatever was causing his suffering. And gradually, over time, this space grew wider, so that it no longer troubled him.

HABIT RELEASER: WATCH THE SKY FOR A WHILE

Pain and suffering can be likened to the weather, while your awareness can be seen as the sky. Sometimes the weather is wild and wintry. Other times it is calm, clear and sunny. But no matter what happens to the weather, the sky always remains.

One of the best ways of gaining a sense of this simple but profound idea is to simply watch the sky for a while. So each day this week, go outside and watch the sky for fifteen minutes (or longer if you wish). If you can't go outside, try looking out of the window instead. And if you can't see the sky for any reason, then spend the time imagining the movement of clouds across the sky in your mind's eye.

It does not matter whether the sky is clear and sunny or grey and overcast. It is always full of shifting patterns, even if they are not apparent at first. If it is cloudy, watch how the clouds drift across the sky. Do they move fast or slowly? Do the clouds bubble up and grow or slowly evaporate? Do they have rounded edges or long tendrils? Do they build up in the sky like enormous mountains or spread thinly outwards? How does their colour vary from region to region and from moment to moment? Simply observe without judgement.

Do the patterns of thought in your mind behave in a similar way? Pause for a moment and observe your own mind at work. Do your thoughts, feelings and emotions possess great power and momentum, while at other times they simply bubble away in the background? Do they shift seamlessly between happy and content and anxious and depressed? Does your pain behave in a similar way? Is it sometimes unbearable, while at others it is hardly noticeable at all?

Turning your awareness back to the sky, if it appears impenetrably grey, watch how the colour varies from one moment to the next and from horizon to horizon. No cloudy sky is ever grey. There are always nuances. See how many you can notice.

If it is a warm, sunny day, watch a patch of sky and see if any clouds form. Continue to watch as the cloud decays. Observe a cloud from birth to death. Clouds are remarkable and powerful things, if you pay them full attention. They appear soft and wispy and yet some are strong enough to break the wings off an airliner.

If it's a clear blue sky with no clouds, can you see any birds soaring on thermals? Or perhaps dust and litter? Can you see the moon – or even a few stars? It is surprising how often the moon can be seen, even on the sunniest of days.

Bring your attention back to yourself. Is your awareness like the sky you've been watching? Is your pain like the clouds – sometimes here and sometimes not? Pause for a while and soak up this expanded awareness. There's no rush to get back to daily life. You can stay here as long as you wish.

CHAPTER SIX

Week Three: Learning to Respond, Rather than React

Once there was a woodcutter in a far-off kingdom. One day he was sent into a wild forest to cut down all of the trees for a new fleet of ships. He frantically set to work and chopped down tree after tree with his steely axe. For weeks on end he huffed and puffed as he cut down the trees, pausing only rarely to eat a few morsels of food and to mop his brow.

One day, a wise old woman arrived and watched him silently for a while.

'What do you want, old crone?' the woodcutter asked.

'Why are you working so hard?' she replied. 'Wouldn't it be faster and easier if you took a little time to sharpen your axe?'

'Don't be ridiculous, old woman,' the woodcutter replied. 'Can't you see how many trees I have to cut down today? I don't have time to sharpen my axe!'

How often have you behaved like the woodcutter in this story? Trying to cope with a chronic health condition is such an all-consuming task that your whole life can be devoured in the attempt. You can become like the woodcutter: trapped and exhausted, with no option but to keep on trying ever harder as your tools become increasingly blunt. All you can do is to try to outrun your suffering, bury it under a pile of distractions and squash it with drugs. Although such tactics may have worked in the past, they have long since hit the point of diminishing returns. Nevertheless, it *is* tempting to keep on trying harder in the hope that they will begin to work once again. But is it always sensible to do this? Or is it wiser to try a different approach?

To really get to grips with your pain, suffering and stress you need to change tack – to learn how to sharpen your axe. Week Three helps you do this by introducing a new way in which to manage your pain – and a new meditation to gradually soothe your suffering.

The first two weeks of the mindfulness programme revealed the subtle interplay between mind and body. By now you will have noticed that the mind tends to create tension in the body. This, in turn, enhances pain and suffering. Much of this suffering dissolves when you pay it full mindful attention, but it returns once your mind begins to wander again. Nevertheless, you might have now glimpsed, perhaps for the first time in years, the possibility of a pain-free life. You might have noticed other benefits too. Many people become a little quicker to laugh and slower to anger. Bitterness and sadness gradually dissolve. Day-to-day life becomes less frantic. These are all signs of growing mindful awareness.

During your meditations, have you noticed the influence

that the breath has on the entire body? The breath does not create movement solely in the chest and abdomen: no corner of the body is left untouched by its ceaseless flowing movement. In previous chapters we learned that a free-flowing breath softly massages the back, chest and abdomen. This directly stimulates the immune and nervous systems to promote healing. It gently stretches and realigns the muscles, tendons, ligaments, bones and joints. A free-flowing breath also cleanses these areas of toxins by lightly massaging the body's lymphatic system. Many people report that simply breathing freely – without fear or worry – and focusing on the breath as they do so, has a significant benefit to overall health and wellbeing. Pain and tension evaporate. The breath is life on so many different levels.

This week's practices take their cue from the breath and its ceaseless flowing movement. Over the next week, we suggest that you continue with the Body Scan meditation. To complement its benefits, the Mindful Movement meditation is introduced. Working with your stress and pain on a more physical level is important, as is avoiding the 'boom-and-bust' cycle of over-taxing yourself one day and being incapable of doing anything the next. To this end, this week we also ask you to keep a short diary of your daily tasks and activities. This is the first stage of learning to pace activities throughout your day. In the long run, such 'pacing' will play a vital role in minimising your suffering and promoting overall health and wellbeing. You can see this as akin to finding your own 'mindfulness rhythm'.

Practices for Week Three

- Ten minutes of the Body Scan meditation (see page 63; track 1 on the CD), to be carried out on six days out of the next seven.
- Ten minutes of the Mindful Movement meditation (see page 110, track 3 of the CD) to be carried out on six days out of the next seven. This should ideally be done at a different time of day from the Body Scan meditation. However, if you choose, you can also do an extra Body Scan or Breathing Anchor immediately before the Mindful Movement meditation to help settle your mind and body.
- Begin to keep a pacing diary (see page 122).
- A Habit Releaser: watch a kettle boil (see page 127).

MINDFUL MOVEMENT

If you have lived with pain, illness or stress for some time, you will find the gentle free-flowing movements of the Mindful Movement meditation especially useful. Over the months and years, you may have become less mobile – or even scared of moving – for fear of hurting yourself further. While this is perfectly understandable, it tends to create problems of its own. The human body is designed to move, so remaining still for too long can lead to many secondary health problems. Lack of exercise causes lethargy, nausea, aches, pains and general 'fugginess'. Even feelings of stress and depression can be brought on by remaining still for too long.

The 'exercises' in the Mindful Movement programme are different from ones you may have tried in the past. Firstly, they are not exercises in the traditional sense. The aim is not to stretch as far as possible or to maintain a position for as long as you can. They are not designed primarily to enhance fitness and flexibility, although they will have these benefits in the long run. Rather, they emphasise the quality of awareness you bring to them as you carry them out. We ask you to rest your consciousness deep inside your body, so that you bring a kindly awareness to your movements. In a sense, they simply extend the breath into a wider exercise. You can see them as breath in action. Or as a moving meditation.

Performing mindful movements

Before you begin, you might like to watch a short video demonstration of the exercises and how to set up your posture (you will find them on www.breathworks-mindfulness.org.uk and http://franticworld.com/resources/). These videos are for guidance only. It's best to carry out the practices themselves while listening to track 3 on the audio CD, as this will enhance the meditative aspects of the movements.

Posture

The Mindful Movements can be performed either sitting or standing. At the start of each exercise, we will suggest the most suitable posture. However, you should always work within your own physical constraints, so please adopt whatever position is the most comfortable for you. If you find any of the exercises too challenging, adapt them to suit your own needs. Try to become sensitive to your body's movements. See them as an expression of the rhythm of the breath. If your fitness and flexibility are limited, be careful not to push yourself too far. Instead, progressively enhance your range of movement. Always bear in mind that it is the quality of awareness you bring to the movements that is paramount. If you are unable to carry out some of the exercises, try visualising yourself carrying them out in your mind's eye. Research shows that this too can improve your fitness and health.[1]

Safety

This week's exercises have been developed over many years with the help of thousands of patients, so they are safe to carry out. Nevertheless, you might like to discuss them with your doctor, specialist or physiotherapist, and practise them with care, leaving out any that you – or they – feel are unsuitable for your illness, injury or disability. Try to avoid the trap of believing that you 'should' be able to move in a certain way – or to a certain extent. Forcing yourself to meet your preconceptions can lead to injury. Instead, try to inhabit your body mindfully, with kindly awareness and curiosity. Even the smallest movement can be surprisingly fulfilling and beneficial.

Hard and soft edges

Try to strike a balance between pushing yourself too far and not stretching yourself enough. This can be tricky, so aim to become aware of your own character when it comes to exercise. If you tend to push yourself, then pay attention to this temptation as you move – and perhaps back off a little. If exercise tends to alarm or frighten you, then see if you can ask a little more of yourself.

How do you strike such a balance? A good way is to try to work within your 'hard' and 'soft' edges. So when you bend your knee, for example, the soft edge is the point at which you first feel a sensation of stretch and compression. Finding the soft edge requires sensitivity, so work slowly and mindfully. Gently probe your sensations. When you feel a stretch or a challenge, move a little deeper into the movement with the help of the breath. Move only a *little* deeper into the movement – and no further.

If you go too far, you'll reach the 'hard' edge. This is the last point of movement before a strain or injury occurs. You'll know that you've passed the hard edge when it feels as if you've begun forcing the movement. You might even start to tremble a little.

Working between these hard and soft edges is ideal. It means that your body is being mobilised without strain. The most creative place to work is a moderate stretch that can be sustained, not an intense one that you can't hold for long. It's also worth bearing in mind that your edges will change as you grow stronger and more flexible. They may change from day to day as well.

Different sorts of pain to watch out for

It can be hard to distinguish between the healthy aches and pains that signify progress and those which indicate that you have pushed yourself too far. A dull ache, muscle tiredness or sensations of stretch are natural and lessen over time. If you notice 'electrical', 'nervy' or sharp sensations, you should reduce the range of the movement or, if it becomes too intense, you should stop for the day. It's sensible to err on the side of caution; you can always carry on tomorrow. Mindful Movements are a journey, not a destination. So there is no rush. And remember: you can always check with your health professional if you have any concerns.

Try to remember

- As best you can, aim to adopt an attitude of play and curiosity. See if you can drop into a deep awareness of the breath as you move, allowing it to lead the pace of the movement, rather than forcing it or rushing through them.
- If you're working with an injury, it's usually helpful to do the less challenged parts of your body first.
- Practising the movements regularly can bring surprising progress, even if you seem to be doing very little in any one session.
- Always leave a few minutes at the end of a session to relax completely in a comfortable position. Give your mind and body time to assimilate the effects.

The movements in this book are taken from a more substantial mindful movement programme developed by Breathworks. These include a range of sequences performed lying down, as well as others done sitting or standing (for more information visit www.breathworks-mindfulness.org.uk).

Mindful Movement meditation

If you are sitting, choose a straight-backed chair with a firm base, something like a dining-room chair. Make sure the pelvis is in a neutral position, neither rolling forwards nor backwards, and that your spine is upright, following its natural curves. If you are standing, have your feet hip width apart with your knees soft.

Relax your body into gravity, giving your weight up to the floor or to the chair. Drop your awareness deep in the body.

Wrist rotations

Let your shoulders be relaxed, dropping away from your ears. Breathe as naturally as you can. Gently support one forearm with the opposite hand in a very light hold and gently and smoothly rotate the hand around the wrist in a circle, within your range of movement. Be careful not to overgrip the arm or tense the face, shoulders or belly. Keep the breath soft and even. After you've done a few rotations, turn your wrist in the other direction for a few circles.

Now relax back down into the starting position for a few breaths and notice the effect of the movement, comparing the two sides of the body. Does the side you have just moved feel different from the other? A little more alive, perhaps? Or even a little 'stretched' or perhaps warmer? Notice any sensations you feel in your body. And if you don't observe any particular difference between the two sides of the body, don't worry. Just be aware of that.

Now repeat on the other side. Rest the forearm in the opposite hand and then smoothly rotate the hand around the wrist for a few circles, always checking that the face is soft, the belly is soft, the shoulders are soft, and that the hand holding the forearm is not gripping too tightly. And then reverse direction for a few rotations. At the end, relax your arms back down so they hang loosely at the sides of your body, and shake your arms and hands a little, relaxing the shoulders. Then come back to stillness – having your arms hanging lightly at the sides of the body if you are standing, or resting on your lap if you are sitting, as you feel the effects of the movement.

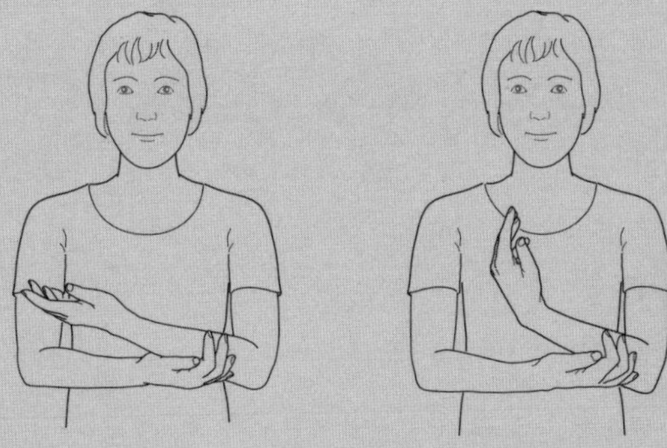

Finger flicking

Before beginning, check that your pelvis is still in neutral – that it's not rolling backwards or forwards – and that the spine is gently upright, following its natural curves. When you're ready, raise one hand up in front of the body and join the thumb and index finger of this raised hand together so they form a circle. Then flick them apart, so they lightly snap out. And now go through each of the other fingers, perhaps repeating several times with each finger. Move and flick each finger lightly and gently, keeping the breathing soft. It's always good to check if you're holding the breath, as we often tend to do so in these kinds of movements. If you notice that you are holding the breath, just relax it again and see if you can bring softness to the face, belly and whole body as you flick the fingers.

Now relax the hand back down and notice if the side you have moved feels different from the other. Be curious, without judgement.

Now repeat the movement with the other hand – raising it up, forming a light circle with the thumb and index finger and then lightly flicking them apart. Do this a few times with the thumb and index finger and then with each of the other fingers in turn. Now repeat the exercise with both hands at the same time. Keep the shoulders relaxed, the face soft, the belly soft, the buttocks soft. At the end, allow the arms to hang loosely on the sides of the body, shaking them a little before coming back to rest. Feel the effects of the movement as you give the weight of your body up to the floor, and let the breath drop deep into the body.

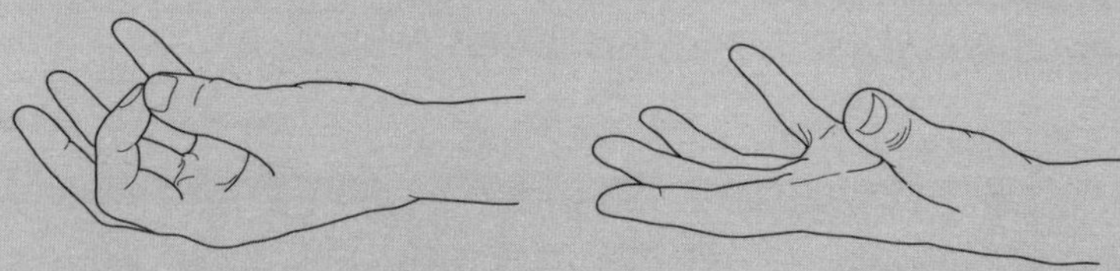

Warm, hugging arms

Start with the arms hanging loosely at the sides of the body. Before moving, tune into the breath for a few moments. On the in-breath, extend both arms at the sides of the body, so the hands come up to shoulder level with the palms facing forwards. As you

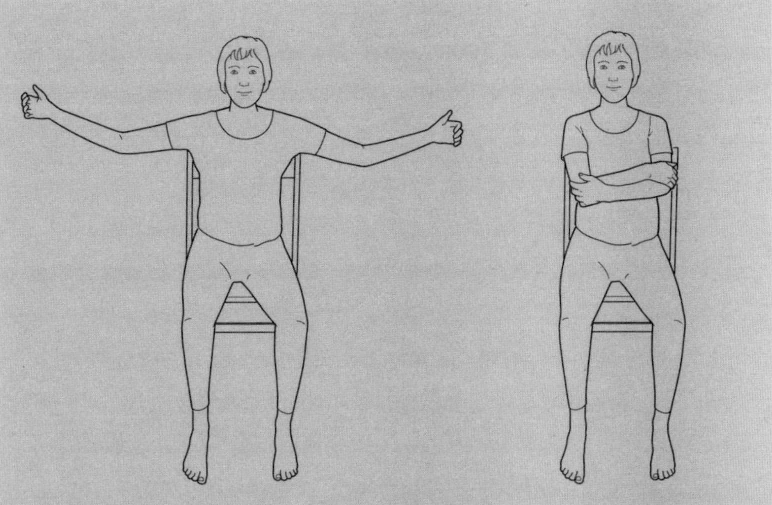

breathe out, very gently draw both arms across your chest, crossing the arms and giving yourself a very gentle hug. Imagine the hug is saturated with warmth and care. On the next in-breath, open the arms again, and on the next out-breath give yourself a hug again. Continue within your own range of movement making the movement quite small if necessary. And you can alternate which arm is on top when you give yourself the hug. As your arms open, feel a corresponding opening in the chest, with the shoulder blades very gently drawing together in the upper back. And as you give yourself a hug with the arms crossed, feel how the upper back broadens and opens. This is a good movement for very gently massaging the spine. Check that the shoulders stay as relaxed as possible as you do this movement. And allow the pace of the movement to be dictated by the rhythm of the natural breath, neither rushing nor holding the breath. After a few hugs, come back to rest. Let the hands hang loosely at the sides of the body and give them a little shake. Feel the effects of the movement. Give your weight up to the floor, letting yourself rest downwards into gravity whether you are sitting or standing. Feel the breath in your whole body.

Peeling off a top

Once again, start with your arms hanging loosely at the sides of the body and tune into the breath for a few moments. Then, on the in-breath, extend both arms up so that the hands are in line with your shoulders with the palms facing downwards, keeping your shoulders relaxed (see opposite, top). As you breathe out, cross your arms in front of the body like the hug. On the next in-breath, imagine you're peeling off a top with both hands, raising the crossed arms up over your head (see opposite, bottom). On the next out-breath, allow your arms to float down the sides of the body with the palms facing downwards, back to the starting position. Repeat this movement a few times in a flowing rhythm, allowing the pace to be dictated by the natural breath. Let your whole spine be massaged very gently by this movement with the chest and back flexing and expanding in the different phases. When you've completed a few cycles, come back to rest. Gently shake the fingers, hands, arms, wrists, elbows and shoulders at the sides of the body before allowing them to come back to stillness. Feel the effects of the movement as you give your weight to the earth beneath you.

Conclusion

Spend some time resting at the end of your Mindful Movement session. You can do this sitting quietly or you might prefer to lie down on the floor or on the bed. Allow your body to release

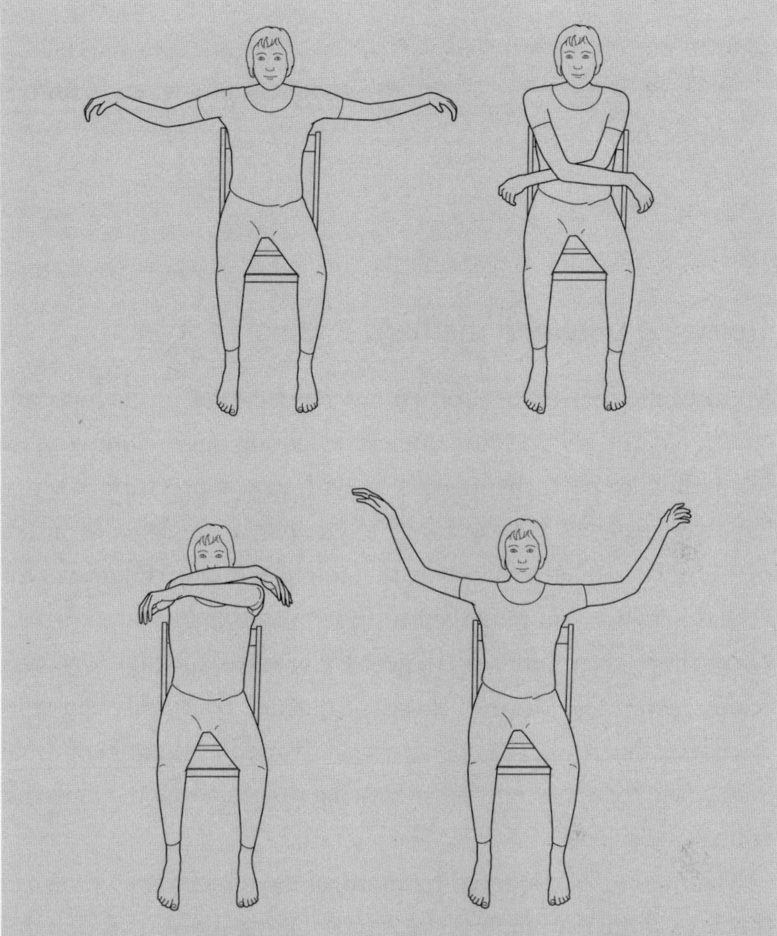

back into stillness and be held and supported by the earth as you feel the effects of the movements. See if you can be sensitive and receptive to all the different sensations in the body: the sensations of the breath and those caused by moving your body. If any are uncomfortable or painful, make sure you include these very gently in your awareness without hardening against them or pushing them away. Allow them to come into being and pass away moment by moment, with a kindly breath. Allow any thoughts, emotions or feelings to come and go without getting caught up in them. When you are ready, begin to move and prepare for the rest of your day.

Tiptoeing between the hard and soft edges

Mindful movement can sometimes release pent-up feelings and emotions. You might find yourself becoming angry with yourself for 'failing' to perform an exercise with expert precision. Or perhaps you feel sad for the range of movement or level of fitness that you've lost. Alternatively, you might feel cheerful and exhilarated because you managed to move more than you expected. Or perhaps the exercises triggered a cascade of long-forgotten happy memories. None of these is unusual. Your body can store memories that are just as poignant and varied as those kept in the mind. And these can end up enhancing or tempering the pain that you actually feel.

The memories triggered by mindful movement can come as a shock to some people. It is the mind's Doing mode in action and it may be the first time in their lives that they have become fully aware of it. The Doing mode, you will recall, is the mind's logical problem-solving state. Have a look back at page 80 for some of its characteristics. It operates by breaking down problems, step by step, into smaller pieces, finding a solution and seeing if it has got you closer to your goal. It works brilliantly at what it does, which is why it volunteers when the mind encounters a problem. Trouble is, when you carry out the Mindful Movement meditation, the mind can interpret the body's stretching sensations as a problem that needs to be solved. It sees the exercises as a challenge and fires up its problem-solving circuits. It wants to make you better by pushing your physical limits. If you were strong and healthy, then this would be a logical thing to do. But if you are not at your physical best, then the Doing mode can end up backfiring by forcing you past the 'hard' edge and beyond. But not only that, as the Doing mode senses your struggling and striving, the mind can dredge up memories of when it felt similarly under pressure in the past. It may bring back memories of the accident or illness that caused your current problems. Or it may rake up fears, worries or memories from your job or private life.

'The first time it happened,' says William, 'I felt slightly overwhelmed. I remembered the bike accident. Then I whispered to myself, "thinking, thinking" and "worrying, worrying". I took a long, deep breath and carried on. I could feel my mind become clear and focused. I then continued with the rest of the exercises.'

By breathing deeply and focusing on the breath, William made a conscious effort to switch his mind into the Being mode. This, you will recall, is the state of mind that allows you to relate directly to the world without your thoughts, feelings and preconceptions acting as a distorting lens. It is not better or worse than the Doing mode, just different.

The Doing mode of mind can be a frequent visitor to these exercises, which, paradoxically, is good news. Each time you catch your mind wandering – drifting into the Doing mode – is another opportunity to practise bringing your awareness back into the body. It may seem like you are failing when you've caught your mind wandering for the umpteenth time, but it is, in fact, a moment of insight. Treasure it. It is your teacher. These moments will gradually dissolve not only your physical pain, but your mental anguish too.

Victoria found it particularly difficult to pick a path between the hard and soft edges. She often went careering past the hard edge and into outright pain. This was buried deep in her character – she was once a mountain marathon runner who was used to pushing her physical limits. Being kind to herself was not in her nature. Nevertheless, by using the breath as a guide she learned to change that. As she breathed out, she would very slightly 'lean' into the movement. And as she did so, Victoria would pay very close attention to the sensations in her body, so that she could sense when she passed over the soft edge and into the middle zone between the two edges. When Victoria breathed in, she would very slightly relax 'back' from the edge. Once again, she would pay close attention to the soft edge and feel herself pass back over it. In this way, she learned to gradually extend her range of movement without pain and began regaining some of her long-lost fitness.

Alison had the opposite reaction to the hard and soft edges. She had become fearful of any pain. As a consequence, when she felt the normal sense of stretching and tightness before she reached the soft edge, she would back off prematurely. After several sessions she decided to 'bite the bullet', as she put it, and pay close attention to the sensations. Alison soon realised that the sensations were not as unpleasant as she feared they would be. In fact, she quite enjoyed the sense of tautness in her muscles. This gave her the courage to approach and pass over the soft edge.

At this point you may be thinking that the Mindful Movement meditation is an extremely tough thing to do. It generally isn't. We have focused on these aspects of it only to give you a sense of the potential difficulties and to provide guidance should you encounter them. Most people enjoy the exercises and gain great benefit and pleasure from them.

MINDFULNESS IN DAILY LIFE – OVERCOMING BOOM AND BUST

Victoria did not only have difficulty picking a path between the hard and soft edges of her mindful movements, she had similar problems in daily life too. As she freely admits, she had a 'boom-and-bust mentality' – an attitude she shares with many other people suffering from chronic illnesses.

'Whenever the pain of my arthritis began to subside I'd begin to push myself a little harder,' says Victoria. 'I'd go for a walk and catch up on the housework. I'd be so happy whenever I had loads of energy to spare. It seemed a shame to not use it all up. The trouble is, I'd wake up the next day completely exhausted and aching all over. Sometimes I'd be in agony. I'd have to double up on the painkillers and feel groggy all day. Sometimes I couldn't get out of bed. It would take me days, sometimes weeks, to get over it. It felt like I was trapped. It just kept happening over and over again. Every time I felt a little better, I'd get on with normal life again. But each time I did so, I'd burn out and end up even less fit and in more pain. There seemed to be no way out. This made me stressed and sometimes depressed too. All I wanted to do was become a little more physically active, but it just didn't seem possible, no matter what I did.'

Victoria's boom-and-bust cycle was entirely natural. Who wouldn't want to get their life back on track when their pain evaporated and vitality returned? Equally, who wouldn't want to crawl away and hide when the pain came back and their energy levels plummeted? Every twist and turn of the boom-and-bust cycle further enhances pain and saps energy. To make matters worse, each twist of the cycle further erodes fitness because you are simply not getting the exercise you need to stay happy and healthy. But it can be even worse than this. You can begin to fear normal day-to-day tasks, lest you hurt yourself once again. All this means, of course, that when vitality returns, the whole cycle begins anew – but this time from an even lower baseline. It's almost as if the very foundations of your life are being slowly eaten away.

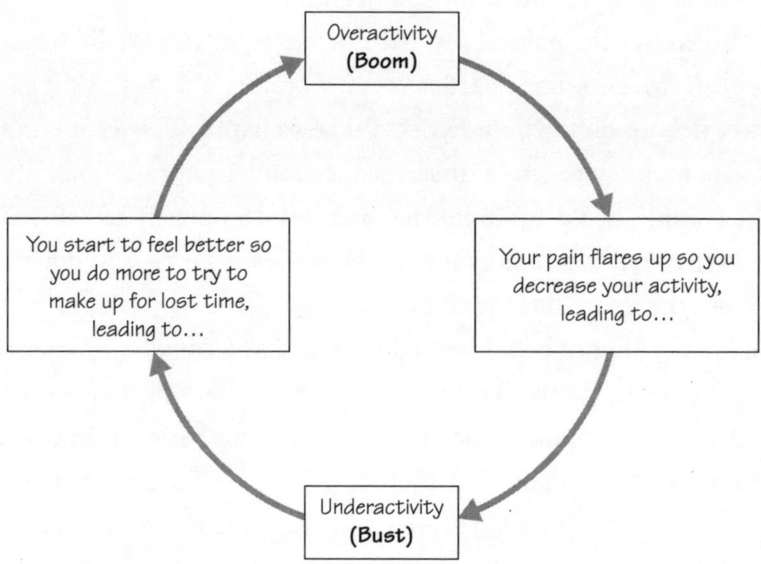

Over time, the amount you can do gradually gets less and less – every time you 'boom' you find you have lost a little bit more fitness, and each time you 'bust' you find yourself sinking lower. Eventually, your capacity for overall fitness declines dramatically.

You can all too easily become trapped in a boom-and-bust cycle when you stop paying attention to the messages that your body is sending you. And the only way out of such a trap is to reconnect with your body once again. Mindfulness is the way out of this trap and it works by allowing you to sense when you are bumping up against your mental and physical limits. It grants you the space to pause – and to back off a little – so that you don't burn out. It works in an equal and opposite way too: it damps down your fears and worries about taking *any* exercise and gives you the motivation to carry out your normal day-to-day activities with renewed vigour. In short, it puts you back in charge of your life and ensures that you are no longer on the back foot living in fear. Mindfulness helps you to gradually peel away the layers of distorted thinking about your experiences, and such reactive feelings as fear, anxiety, stress and despair. Simply put, mindfulness teaches you how to pace yourself. And it's an approach that is widely recommended by pain-management clinics around the world.

The programme detailed below is a simple way of 'pacing' yourself using mindfulness. It involves three steps:

- Firstly, you keep a diary of everything you do for seven days, noting the duration of each activity and its impact on your pain, stress or other symptoms.

- Secondly, you analyse the diary and work out how long you can perform each activity for without causing your pain or symptoms to worsen. These are called your baselines.

- Thirdly, these baselines are gradually lengthened to improve your overall fitness and stamina without tipping you into another boom-and-bust cycle.

Over the coming weeks you will be asked to implement this three-step programme. Although it might appear to be best suited to those suffering from chronic pain and illness, pacing works equally well for stress. After all, stress is a form of mental pain that has many of the same underlying driving forces as physical suffering. Stress can also be aggravated by day-to-day physical activities. Rushing through the housework or frantically typing on the computer at work can conjure up stressful feelings.

This week you should begin keeping a diary – or log – of the main things that you do each day. Next week you will be asked to analyse the diary so that you can create a personalised pacing programme. In subsequent weeks we will help you optimise the scope and tempo of your daily activities. Over time, this will substantially reduce your suffering and stress as well as improving overall fitness. If this sounds a little difficult, don't worry. It isn't. The point of the programme is to establish a comfortable baseline from which you can build. You will *never* be asked to do anything that is too difficult for you to do.

The Pacing Programme: keeping a diary

Over the next seven days keep a detailed log or diary of your daily activities. The aim is to take note of those that tend to aggravate your condition, those that ease it, and those that have no impact at all. A template for the diary can be found in the Appendix (see page 256). Feel free to photocopy it as many times as you need. You can also find templates available to download at www.breathworks-mindfulness.org.uk. A few sample pages from a completed diary can be found on pages 124–6 and at www.franticworld.com. You should complete the entries as follows:

1. Note how long each activity takes and the levels of pain or stress that you feel when you've completed it. Use a scale of zero to ten, where zero is equivalent to no pain or stress, while ten is the worst imaginable. If your difficulty is something other than pain or stress – for example, fatigue or depression – then score this instead.

2. In the right-hand column note whether the pain, stress (or other difficulty you are scoring) is made worse (+), eased (-) or unaffected by the activity (0). Also note rest periods (R).

3. There's also a column for muscle tension. It is useful to see the connection between muscular tension and other symptoms such as aches, pains, feelings of anxiety, stress, depression or exhaustion.

Try to remember to fill in this diary for seven days. Its purpose is to encourage you think about your life, so use column headings that will be most helpful.

You should aim to approach the Pacing Programme like a detective, observing yourself with a kindly eye to see how you spend your time. You should also approach this task with as much of a spirit of kind-hearted awareness as you can muster. Try to remember not to criticise yourself in any way. For example, if you feel that you 'should' be more active, then try not to punish yourself. Instead, try to accept your current physical state for the time being. The aim is simply to establish a baseline from which you can build your fitness, not to create a new whip with which to beat yourself.

Daily activity diary example sheets

Date 25th April					
Time	**Activity**	**Time taken**	**Pain at end** (or whatever symptom you are scoring) **(1–10)**	**Tension at end (1–10)**	**0** (no change in pain or symptom) **+** (increase in pain or symptom) **–** (decrease in pain or symptom) **R** (rest)
9:00–9:30	wake up, have cup of tea and get dressed	30 m	4	4	
–10:00	breakfast – sit up	30 m	5	6	+
–12:00	work at desk	2 hrs	6	6	+
–12:20	meditate – sit	20 m	5	5	–
–12:40	continue meditating – lying	20 m	4	4	–
–13:00	mindful movement	20 m	4	4	0
–14:00	lunch sitting with friend	1 hr	6	5	+
–14:40	body scan	40 m	4	3	–
–16:00	drive to shops, go round supermarket and drive back home	1 hr 20 m	6	7	+
–17:00	rest	1 hr	5	4	R
–18:00	work at desk	1 hr	6	6	+
–19:00	dinner – sitting up	1 hr	7	6	+
– 21:00	watch DVD lying on sofa	2 hrs	5	4	–
–21:30	have a bath	30 m	4	3	–
–22:00	prepare for bed	30 m	5	4	+
–23:00	read until sleep at 23:00	1 hr	5	4	0

Date 26th April					
Time	**Activity**	**Time taken**	**Pain at end** (or whatever symptom you are scoring) **(1–10)**	**Tension at end (1–10)**	**0** (no change in pain or symptom) **+** (increase in pain or symptom) **–** (decrease in pain or symptom) **R** (rest)
8:00 – 8:30	wake up, cup of tea	30 m	5	4	
-9:00	breakfast – sit up	30 m	6	6	+
-9:30	shower and dress	30 m	6	6	0
-11:30	work at desk	2 hrs	7	8	+
-12:30	rest	1 hr	4	4	R
-13:00	meditate – sit	30 m	5	5	+
-14:00	lunch	1 hr	6	5	+
-14:20	body scan	20 m	4	3	–
-16:20	go for swim	2 hrs	6	7	+
-17:30	rest	1 hr 10 m	5	4	R
-19:00	work at desk	1 hr 30 m	7	5	+
-20:00	dinner – sitting up	1 hr	7	6	0
- 21:00	rest and read	1 hr	5	4	- (R)
-21:20	facebook etc on computer	20 m	6	6	+
-22:00	rest and read	40 m	5	4	+
-22:30	prepare for bed	30 m	6	5	+
-23:00	read until sleep at 23:00	30 m	5	4	0

Date 27th April					
Time	**Activity**	**Time taken**	**Pain at end** (or whatever symptom you are scoring) **(1–10)**	**Tension at end (1–10)**	**0** (no change in pain or symptom) **+** (increase in pain or symptom) **–** (decrease in pain or symptom) **R** (rest)
8:00–8:30	wake up, cup of tea	30 m	6	5	
-8:45	few stretches and mindful movements	15 m	5	5	–
-9:30	meditate sitting up (too long!)	45 m	7	7	+
-10:00	shower and dress	30 m	6	6	–
-10:30	breakfast – lying down	30 m	5	5	–
-11:30	work at desk	1 hr	6	6	+
-12:10	phone call to mum	40 m	5	5	–
-13:00	work at desk	50 m	6	6	+
-14:00	lunch	1 hr	5	5	–
-14:20	body scan	20 m	4	3	–
-17:20	rest	3 hrs	4	4	R
-17:50	short walk	30 m	7	5	+
-19:00	work at desk	1 hr 10 m	7	6	0
-20:00	dinner	1 hr	6	5	–
-22:00	watch TV – lying down	2 hrs	5	4	–
-22:30	prepare for bed	30 m	6	5	+
-23:00	read until sleep at 23:00	30 m	5	4	0

HABIT RELEASER: WATCH A KETTLE BOIL

Boiling a kettle of water is one of those things that we all do several times each day without a moment's thought. So at least once per day, every day this week, try paying full mindful attention to filling and boiling a kettle of water.

As you lift the kettle to fill it, how heavy does it feel? Do you fill it via the spout or do you open the lid? Is the lid stiff? Pay full attention as the water swills out of the tap and into the kettle. Does it hiss and bubble? Does it smell? We are so accustomed to the smell of water that we no longer notice it. Try to imagine how strong the smell of moisture would be if you'd just spent a week in a desert. Spend a few moments thinking about how the water reached you. The rain falling on the distant mountains, trickling through rock and soil, until it eventually reaches a stream. Imagine the reservoir, the water-treatment works, the pipelines. Now imagine all of the engineers and maintenance workers who designed, built and maintained the water network. Think of the people involved in producing and distributing the electricity; the people growing and distributing the tea, coffee or cocoa that you will use to make your drink. We are all interconnected on a myriad of levels. And this is just for a cup of tea.

As you return the kettle to the work surface or cooker, pay close attention to your own movements. Were you aware of those movements or did they 'just happen'? Likewise, did you consciously flick the electric switch to 'On' or light the cooker – or did the autopilot take care of things?

Now listen as the kettle begins to heat. What can you hear? Close your eyes and drink up the sounds. Check in with yourself. What mode of mind are you operating in? After a few moments, see if you can notice the first stirrings of impatience. Where in the body are they to be found? What do they feel like? Do they feel like a force trying to break out and exert control? Habits of impatience can be compelling.

When the kettle is almost boiled, what do you do? Do you wait until the thermostat clicks off – or do you rush in and pour the water before it's boiled? See if you can be patient and wait for the thermostat to click off before mindfully lifting the kettle, being aware of your breath and pouring the water.

Spend a moment considering if there are other aspects of daily life that can also be used to cultivate mindfulness. Such 'everyday mindfulness' can be at least as important as the formal meditations.

Now take your cup of tea, coffee or cocoa and relax. You've earned it.

CHAPTER SEVEN

Week Four: Watching Your Suffering and Stress Dissolve

Shortly after the British mountaineer George Mallory died while attempting to climb Everest in 1924, a journalist asked why the team had continued with their assault on the summit on that fateful day.

'The price of life is death,' replied one of the survivors.

That single sentence sums up the human condition more than any other. We are here on this earth for a short while, we experience a panoply of bittersweet emotions, and then depart. We forget this at our peril.

Virtually all of us avoid thinking about pain, suffering and death as much as we can, for as long as we can, usually until it is too late. While this is entirely natural, it carries a high but largely hidden price. For if we cannot face up to life's difficulties, then we cannot deal with them effectively. Such aversion enhances pain and suffering, closes down the mind and leaves behind a deep-seated sense of fear and caution. And paradoxically, by not facing up to difficulties we run the risk of dulling our awareness to all that is wonderful about life, in all of its tingling beauty.

Whenever we're faced with a difficulty – whether it's pain, illness or stress – it's only natural to try to push it away. We can do this in myriad ways, such as endlessly churning through previously failed solutions, ignoring it or burying it under a pile of distractions. But sooner or later, there comes a point where these strategies no longer work and either we run out of steam or the difficulty we're facing becomes truly overwhelming. When we reach this fork in the road, we have two options. We can try to carry on, pretending that nothing is wrong (and lead an increasingly impoverished existence), or we can embrace a different way of relating to ourselves and the world. This different approach is one of mindful acceptance of ourselves and of our suffering. It means turning towards it, accepting it, even if we hate it, or it fills us with fear and dread.

For many of us, especially those who live with chronic pain or stress, the idea of 'acceptance' is pure heresy. It smacks of passively accepting your fate. Why should you 'give up' and live without hope? But mindful acceptance demands none of these things. The flavour of acceptance that arises from the full conscious awareness engendered by mindfulness is subtly different from the usual passive form of acceptance. In the context of mindfulness, acceptance is simply a pause, a period of allowing, of letting be, of clear seeing. It is an acceptance that this is the way things are, for now. It is about embracing life, not merely tolerating it.

Mindful acceptance has another strand too: one of compassion towards others and the world around you. We'll be exploring this more fully in later chapters, but the first step is learning to be compassionate towards yourself. This requests that you to stop attacking yourself for your perceived 'failures', 'weaknesses' and 'inadequacies'. It asks that you stop blaming yourself for your predicament. Most of all, it encourages you to gently allow yourself to be just as you are, with all of your faults and foibles, your aches and pains. For some, this can be harder than coping with pain, suffering and stress. In the long run, though, compassionate acceptance will dramatically reduce pain and improve your life.

Many scientific studies show the power of compassionate acceptance; it dissolves all the stresses, fears and worries that lie before it. And, crucially, just like the other benefits of mindfulness, these changes become hard-wired into the brain. Scans show significant positive changes in the parts of the brain associated with raw emotion and the perception of pain. And, remarkably, these physical changes begin to appear after just eight weeks of practising meditations such as Compassionate Acceptance.[1] Then, over time, when pain does appear, it is less intense than in the past and fades away again more quickly. Anxiety, stress, depression and exhaustion occur less often too and with lower intensity. So it becomes progressively easier to face the world with a calm, compassionate and accepting state of mind. It's a virtuous cycle.

This week you will begin learning how to turn towards the heart of your pain and suffering. You may find it difficult – not because of what you will find, but because of what you *fear* you will find. For this reason, some people consider abandoning the programme at this point. If you are tempted to do so, please remember that although our programme may not feel easy, it is better than the alternative, which is to continue living a life marred by suffering and stress. If you should feel any fear or trepidation, try to remember that all of the effort that you have put into carrying out the programme so far has been leading up to this point. You have built up your powers of concentration and learned how to reconnect your mind and body. You have set the stage. Now it is time to begin using your new-found skills to substantially improve your life.

Practices for Week Four

- Ten minutes of the Breathing Anchor meditation (see page 92; track 2 on the CD), to be carried out on six days out of the next seven.
- Ten minutes of the Compassionate Acceptance meditation (see page 134; track 4 on the CD), to be carried out on six days out of the next seven (ideally at a different time of day from the Breathing Anchor meditation). You can also do extra meditations, such as the Body Scan, immediately before the Compassionate Acceptance meditation to help you settle.
- Analyse your pacing diary and begin to implement your 'baselines' (see page 144 and 147).
- A Habit Releaser: make peace with gravity (see page 154).

ACCEPTANCE

One of the central teachings of the Breathworks programme is distinguishing between the two elements of suffering: Primary and Secondary. Primary Suffering is the actual unpleasant sensations felt in your body in any given moment; Secondary

Suffering is the additional pain that arises when you resist and react against this experience. Secondary Suffering is often a greater source of distress than the actual sensations of pain in the body. And as you are learning first-hand, mindfulness training helps you to reduce or even completely overcome Secondary Suffering by accepting the primary sensations. This leaves you with far less suffering to actually live with. In essence, you learn to accept the things that you cannot change (the Primary Suffering) and to change those you can (the Secondary Suffering).

Week Four helps you to compassionately turn towards any discomfort that you experience and to feel the raw sensations. You will learn to observe them as their intensity rises and falls and to experience the soothing effects of the breath. You will practise letting go of your habitual reactions when you notice that they've arisen. But most of all, you will learn to sense the difference – at a deep-seated and visceral level – between Primary and Secondary Suffering. In this way, mindfulness can be seen as a middle way between suppressing your feelings on the one hand – blocking them out through fear or avoidance – and over-identifying with them by reacting and drowning in your experiences on the other.

In essence, mindfulness means being clear and honest about your experiences as they arise and then pass away. It teaches you that you do not have to react to your suffering. Nor do you have to resist it. It is this reaction and resistance that drives Secondary Suffering. So if you do not react, most – and possibly all – of your suffering will melt away.

Some people find it difficult to cultivate the 'correct' flavour of compassionate awareness for this meditation; it can turn in on itself, becoming yet another rod with which they beat themselves: *Why can't I even be nice to myself . . . ? I can't even get that right!* If you find that this is the case for you, simply observe your own mind in action for a few moments. This is to gently dissolve your worries, stresses and judgemental ways of thinking. Try not to criticise yourself in any way. Simply accept for this moment that you are worried, stressed or self-critical. Being compassionate towards your own feelings is the best starting point for this meditation.

If you should find yourself concerned about this, simply pause for a while to accept your feelings and smile inwardly to yourself, even if it initially feels a little false. Try bringing to mind someone you love. Or perhaps a favourite pet, even if they have long since departed. Bringing to mind a favourite place can help too. The important thing is to bring to mind a sense of warmth and compassion, however false this may at first appear. You then gently, as well as you can, transfer these feelings to yourself so that you suffuse yourself with warmth, love and compassion.

But please try to remember that you cannot fail at mindfulness, and this applies especially to the Compassionate Acceptance meditation. Your state of mind is your state of mind. If you don't like your current state of mind, simply wait a while – another one will be along in a minute.

Compassionate Acceptance meditation

In this meditation you're going to learn how to very, very gently turn towards your experience of pain or difficulty and to meet it with tenderness, kindness and compassion. This will help to soften or dissolve secondary resistance and suffering. And you'll learn how to bathe your pain or difficulty, as well as any resistance you may feel, in a kindly, tender breath, moment by moment.

Preparation

Establish a comfortable posture – we suggest either sitting or lying if it's comfortable, but you can choose any posture that is suitable for you.

Gently surrender the weight of your body to gravity, so it settles and rests on the bed, the floor or the chair. Can you let go into a sense of how gravity gently draws your body down towards the floor and holds you and supports you?

The Meditation

Gradually gather your awareness around the breath in the whole body, allowing yourself to be rocked and cradled by the breath – the front, the sides and the back of the body. Feel the breath deeply inside. Can you rest your awareness inside the breath as it rhythmically and gently moves the body?

And now, with great tenderness, gently open your awareness to include your pain, discomfort, fatigue or difficulty of whatever kind you're experiencing. Include it in your awareness with the kind of attitude that you would naturally have towards a loved one who was hurting or injured. Softly breathe with this experience for a few moments. If this feels frightening, then breathe with the fear with gentleness, coming back to rest your awareness on the breath in the body, over and over.

If you feel resistant, or your pain feels very hard and stuck, then you may find the following image helpful: picture your resistance and pain as a bale of hay that you're standing or sitting beside. Imagine you're very, very gently leaning against the bale of hay – gradually giving your weight to its surface. As you lean on it, the bale gives a little bit on receiving your weight, and you realise that the surface is more pliable and yielding than you'd thought. Can you get a sense of your resistance towards your pain softening in a similar way to the bale of hay as you 'lean into' it? And all the time your body is gently moving and being rocked with a tender breath.

Now, allowing your awareness to become a little more precise, investigate the exact sensations of pain or discomfort. What do you feel? Do you notice the way the sensations are always changing and how no two moments are precisely the same? And maybe as you come closer to your actual experience, you realise for example, that it's just your lower back that's hurting, rather than your whole back as you'd previously thought. Can you apply this close investigation to whatever your particular difficulty is? And maybe you'll discover that some of the sensations have aspects to them that are pleasant – things like tingling. Or you may even feel a sense of relief in your heart, now that you're finally turning towards your difficulty and meeting it with kindness and curiosity, rather than being locked in battle with it, which just leads to more suffering and tension.

And what about your thoughts and emotions? Are you having any thoughts and emotions about your pain or difficulty? Can you let them come and go moment by moment, neither suppressing them nor over-identifying with them? Can you let them go a little bit as you rest with the basic sensations in the body, moment by moment, held by the kindly breath?

Be sure to cultivate an attitude that is patient, gentle and tender.

If your experience is a little overwhelming, you can broaden your awareness to include other aspects of the moment. Notice sounds, smells, the temperature in the room perhaps; allow your sensations of pain or discomfort to take place within a broad and open field of awareness that includes many things as they arise and pass away.

And if you're feeling a little blocked or numb, you may like to turn towards your experience with a little more focus. Be curious about the actual sensations, thoughts or emotions you're experiencing and soften around them. Use the breath to soften resistance or hardness. Imagine that the breath is very soothing, allowing it to naturally dissolve away resistance and hardness, even if just a tiny bit.

And now saturate the breath with self-compassion: as you breathe in, imagine a sense of kindliness flowing into your whole body; and as you breathe out, imagine the kindness seeping ever deeper, saturating the body with warmth and compassion. Breathe in and out with a deep sense of kindliness, care, tenderness and compassion towards yourself.

Allow the whole body, including any pain or discomfort that may be present, to be rocked and cradled by the breath. And if you still feel dominated by resistance, then allow that to be saturated by the kindly, gentle breath. Accept all of your experience with great tenderness.

Conclusion

Very gently begin to bring this meditation to a close. Expand your awareness to include sounds inside and outside the room. Open your eyes and allow your awareness to remain deep inside your body as you begin to gently move, with an attitude of kindliness and care towards yourself. Then, very gradually, re-engage with the activities of the day, seeing if you can bring this quality of self-compassion with you and allowing kindness to flow into your experience, over and over again. Soften resistance and aversion with a kindly breath, no matter what activity you are engaged with.

Some people find the Compassionate Acceptance meditation a little overwhelming at first. It can feel as if years of accumulated fears and worries have been unleashed at once – like a dam bursting – so it's not surprising that you can feel a little overcome. Michael learned that a good way of dealing with these feelings is to float along with them – like a cork bobbing on the sea – rather than trying to fight or suppress them. He was a lifeguard, so he adapted the approach that he used when rescuing swimmers who had got into difficulty:

'I realised that I was drowning under my pain and emotions,' he says. 'At first I fought like crazy – like the people I used to rescue. But it is impossible to swim against a powerful tide and equally impossible to fight the current of your emotions. You have to be more skilful than that. When you rescue someone from the sea, you first calm their fears and then you begin to swim sideways out of the current. You never fight the current because you will never win.'

Michael learned that he could 'swim sideways' through the current of his emotions by broadening his awareness. He mentally took a step backwards, so that he could sense his whole field of awareness, including the rhythm of his breath, the feel of his clothes on his skin and the sounds of the sea in the background – as well as the pain in his body. In this way, he became a 'bigger container' for the turbulence of his mind and body. And once he'd broadened his consciousness in this way, he realised that he could 'float' on the current of his awareness. He'd gently remind himself that, 'It's OK to feel this. It's OK to be with it.' By doing this he found that, inch by inch, he could bring compassionate acceptance back into his meditation.

'I accepted that it would take a long time to recover from my injuries. That acceptance meant that I was no longer fighting myself, so I began to sleep better, I was less "stressy" and I was able to continue with my physiotherapy. I began to heal so much faster.'

Another way of dealing with a sudden rush of unpleasant sensations is to gently remind yourself that you do not have to deal with everything at once. You can take a step back. You can approach the edge of your pain, and if the feelings become too intense, then you can focus your awareness elsewhere – on the breath perhaps – before returning with a renewed sense of warmth, curiosity and compassion. The aim is not to block the unpleasant sensations or to ignore them, but simply to move your awareness elsewhere for a while. If, after a few moments, you feel sufficiently confident, then you can return your awareness to the difficult sensations. Always try to remember that there is no rush to return. You do not have to feel everything at once. Often, though, when you do return, you will find that the unpleasantness has diminished.

On the other hand, some people experience the opposite of 'drowning' and find that they tend to feel rather numb or cut off from their experience. If this happens to you, you can try moving a little closer to the actual sensations that you are experiencing and investigate their qualities in a little more detail. Are they sharp or smooth? Loud or soft? Jagged or achy? You might also like to investigate their 'nature': observe how they continually change, arising and passing away, moment by moment. They might feel intense one moment and then change to a more pleasurable tingly sensation in the next. In this way, you might discover that your pain or discomfort is not as solid as you thought. You might also find that it is perhaps not as widespread or pervasive as you had at first believed. When you habitually avoid an experience, it can become the centre of your attention, dominating your life – like a monster that lurks around every corner. It can become far worse than the actual moment-by-moment sensations warrant.

It is not just physical experiences that can become numbed or 'blocked'. Emotions can too. Caroline noticed that she tended to avoid her more difficult emotions. This worked for a while, until, that is, they became truly overwhelming. So she often found herself being plunged headlong into severe anxiety attacks. She'd imagine all of the things that could go wrong in the future. Before long she'd be punished by such hellish thoughts as: *'Oh, my God I'm going to die; there's so little time; I'm not making the most of my life; I'm getting it all wrong; there's something wrong with me; I deserve to die . . .'* These bouts of extreme anxiety and stress manifested in her body as physical tension, nausea and fatigue. And these, in turn, fed her fears about her failing health.

Through the Compassionate Acceptance meditation Caroline learned to recognise the individual feelings of anxiety before they grew into what she called her 'emotional disaster'. By recognising the initial feelings of anxiety – by simply feeling and accepting them – unpleasant though it was, she prevented them from snowballing out of control. This was a revelation to her. Gradually, as the weeks passed, Caroline had fewer and fewer 'emotional splurges' and regained her inner confidence.

Victoria described the experience of being overwhelmed by her difficulties as akin to falling over in mud, becoming completely covered in it and then not being able to wash it off. Wherever she went, the mud went with her. It was as if all of her unpleasant life experiences were sticking to her like glue. Through the Compassionate Acceptance meditation, however, she saw how all of this mud was like Secondary Suffering. She discovered that by very gently breathing *with* her suffering and her tormented thoughts she could relax into a more fluid and open state of mind. Gradually, the sense of being caked in mud began to lessen; it was as if the meditation gently washed it off. It came as a revelation when she realised that a lot of the 'mud' was caused by her judging herself for feeling so bad, and for blaming herself with the misguided assumption that she 'should' feel differently. The Compassionate Acceptance meditation meant she could accept everything far more easily.

Flic found it almost impossible to accept her Paget's disease, a metabolic condition that left her with severe pain in her left leg and knee. She was partially crippled and had to use a stick to move even a few metres. There is no 'cure' for the disease and it is treated largely with painkillers that left Flic feeling 'numb' all over.

'I set about trying to find a cure for my pain,' she says. 'I *was determined to* find a solution to this. This desperate seeking only added to my distress. I'd known I was carrying some emotional pain alongside my physical pain, but I hadn't known just how much that was. Being led gently through the meditation with tenderness and kindliness, I was a shocked to see how much resistance I had towards it. My heart felt like a boulder in my chest. How could it hurt so much?

'But facing up to the things that I'd been avoiding for so long, that proved to be my turning point. It wasn't easy at first. I think I wept on and off for nearly a week, but I had a sense of relief too; I could now begin to rest in my body and experience – moment by moment. I could see by trying to avoid difficult emotions, by pushing them away, that I'd been adding layer upon layer of distress. Mindfulness helped me gently dissolve those layers.

'I still live with some physical pain, I still walk with a stick – I accept that this isn't going to change and that's OK. I no longer live with years of accumulated emotional pain. Mindfulness didn't just change my life – mindfulness saved my life.'

Simple acceptance can often trigger a chain of events that radically reduces pain, suffering and stress. Elaine discovered this for herself.

'My discovery of mindfulness has been life-changing. I would say my chronic pain has reduced by approximately 80 to 90 per cent. Honestly – truly – I went from feeling pain each day to feeling twinges once or twice a month, if that. I have also noticed that if I do not take time to practise these simple but life-enhancing mindful techniques, my pain and also my anxiety and stress can begin to increase again.

'I do not think for a minute my pain wasn't real – in the beginning it was very real. I had a bad injury and my body was telling me I needed to slow down, rest, change my lifestyle, get some rehab, etc. Over time, my body began to heal. However, my mind was so used to feeling pain it expected nothing else – the mind is so powerful, it can prove you wrong or prove you right based on what you believe.

'Why should you be mindful and kind to yourself? The pace of life has meant we rarely take time to pause, breathe and relax.

That is no good; no good at all for either our mental or physical health.'

Throughout the Compassionate Acceptance meditation, the best you can, see if you can avoid the temptation to try to 'fix' your pain. Because compassion and acceptance are linked to positive changes it is only natural to want to use them to solve your problems. This is the Doing mode at work. If the Doing mode of mind fires up it will trigger a cascade of events that may, eventually, lead you back into a vicious cycle by activating the mind's autopilot and aversion pathways. This will lead to further tension and stress that will, in turn, fuel your suffering and stress and probably hamper your healing as well. By contrast, consciously shifting gear into the Being mode, which is founded on acceptance and compassion, will progressively lead to tremendously positive changes in your life. Of course, it is not possible to completely eliminate the desire to use this meditation to cure your suffering, so simply be aware of the tendency.

Pete found that by accepting the reality of his Parkinson's disease he could live a far more fulfilling life. After years of struggle he came to an acceptance that there was very little 'fixing' to be done: he had a condition that was likely to become progressively worse. He initially became annoyed and angry with his slowly failing body, but found that introducing kindliness into the breath helped ease his anger, bitterness and stress. It helped him feel more kindness towards himself as he came to terms with his Parkinson's disease. Gradually, he discovered a deep-seated acceptance of his life as it is. He realised he had a very good life despite the fact that he has Parkinson's. As he began to accept his condition, his stress levels lowered and his Parkinson's symptoms became less dominant and troubling.

THE PACING PROGRAMME: ANALYSING YOUR DIARY

Last week we introduced the concept of 'pacing' to help you cope more effectively with daily life. This week we ask you to analyse your pacing diary. This is straightforward and should take only around twenty to thirty minutes. It might be worth making a mental note of when you will do this so you can set aside the time. Don't worry if you feel that your diary is not sufficiently comprehensive. You can continue to keep it for another few days – or for as long as you feel is necessary. Try to remember that the aim is not to produce a 'perfect' diary, but to build up a reasonably comprehensive picture of your daily activities along with the stresses, strains and suffering that they cause. Pacing should be seen as a 'work in progress' and adapted to suit your changing circumstances.

This week we ask you to do two things:

1. Analyse your diary.
2. Establish a 'baseline' for each of your daily activities. This baseline is the amount of time that you can comfortably spend carrying out an activity before it starts to cause undue stress or discomfort. Once established, you can then gradually build on these baselines to optimise your health and well-being.

Although pacing is aimed primarily at relieving pain and illness, it does also work with chronic stress. If you have spent years suffering with chronic stress, you will gain great benefits from learning to pace yourself through the day. It will help you forestall the build-up of tension and thereby gradually defuse your stress.

1. Analysing your diary

You will find a blank analysis sheet in the Appendix (see page 257). You can also find a template available to download at www.breathworks-mindfulness.org.uk or www.franticworld.com. Your first step is to transfer the information from your diary into the three columns of this sheet. Copy as many sheets as you need, either by hand or with a photocopier. An example of a completed sheet is shown overleaf.

Transfer to the '+' column of your analysis sheet those activities that cause extra pain or stress – or any of the other symptoms that you have decided to monitor. In the '0' column record activities that make no difference, and put any that reduce your pain (or other symptoms) into the '-' column. When you transfer the information, also make a note of the amount of time spent on each activity.

You will probably discover that simply transferring the information to the analysis sheet will reveal patterns that you were unaware of. It may even highlight something obvious that immediately improves your condition. For example, you could discover that sitting aggravates your condition, while lying down eases it. This might mean that you need to pace the amount of time you spend sitting to avoid a flare-up.

Steve is a schoolteacher who, for many years, suffered from chronic back pain. When Steve analysed his diary, he discovered that his pain was caused largely by wiping the blackboard. When he stopped, his pain declined virtually to zero.

It is also not unusual for people to discover that they never

Diary analysis example sheet

DIARY EXTRACT (from one whole week's dairies)

+ **Extra Pain** (or whatever symptom you are scoring)	0 **No change in pain** (or whatever symptom you have scored)	– **Reduced pain** (or whatever symptom you have scored)
breakfast – sit up (30 m)	mindful movement (20 m)	lie down to meditate (20 m)
work at desk – sitting (1 hr)	read in bed until sleep (1 hr)	lie down for body scan (40 m)
MEDITATE – SIT (20 m)	shower and dress (30 m)	lie down and watch DVD on sofa (2 hrs)
lunch – sitting with friend (1 hr)	dinner – sitting up (1 hr)	take a bath (30 m)
drive to supermarket, shop, and back home (1 hr 20m)	read in bed until sleep (30 m)	lie down for body scan (20 m)
work at desk – sitting (1 hr)	work at desk (1 hr 10 m)	lie on bed to rest and read (1 hr)
dinner – sitting up (1 hr)	meditation – lying down (40 m)	lie on bed to rest and read (40 m)
prepare for bed (30 m)	take a bath (20 m)	few stretches and mindful movement (15 m)
work at desk – sitting (2 hrs)	lie on bed and read (30 m)	shower and dress (30 m)
meditate – sit (30 m)	cooking (20 m)	lie down for breakfast (30 m)
go for swim (2 hrs)	lie down for phone call (1 hr)	lie down for phone call to mum (40 m)
work at desk – sitting (1 hr 30 m)	potter about in room (45 m)	lie down for lunch (1 hr)
FACEBOOK ETC. ON COMPUTER – SIT (20 m)	drive to shops (30 m)	lie down and watch DVD (1 hr)
meditate – sitting (45 m)		lie down for dinner (1 hr)
work at desk – sitting (50 m)		lie down and watch TV (2 hrs)
short walk (30 m)		lie down in meeting (1 hr)
SIT TO TALK ON PHONE (20 m)		
drive to shops (45 m)	**BASELINE SIT: minimum caused extra pain = 20 mins. 80% = 16 mins**	
LUNCH – SIT (20 m)		

take a break, and so run out of space on the diary sheet. This alone might explain their exhaustion, stress and insomnia.

If you have a condition that means you need to rest a lot, you should also make a note of your rest periods. You might discover that you are resting far more on some days than on others. If this is the case, then you might want to spread out your rest periods. An example of Vidyamala's completed rest period sheet is shown below, and you will a find blank sheet for this in the Appendix (see page 258) (you can also find a template available to download at www.breathworks-mindfulness.org.uk and www.franticworld.com).

Rest period analysis example sheet

Date	Length	Total number	Total time
25th April	1 hr	1	1 hr
26th April	1 hr, 1 hr 10m, 1 hr, 40 m	4	3 hrs 50 m
27th April	3 hrs	1	3 hrs

(You can see from this example that when I examined my diary for the period of the three days outlined on pages 124–6, I discovered the rest periods were very unbalanced. I would not have realised this without keeping the diary.)

Establishing your baselines

Once you have analysed your diary, you are ready to calculate your baselines – the amount of time that you can do an activity for without it causing an increase in pain or other symptoms. You may find that your symptoms vary from day to day, but by establishing a baseline you can set a consistent and steady pace that will not exacerbate them.

To establish a baseline you need to look at the '+' column on your analysis sheet where you have recorded activities that caused your symptoms to increase. Next, identify the shortest time that you spent on each activity. This indicates that even this relatively short period of time is too long. On Vidyamala's example sheet (see page 146), you will see that the minimum amount of time that sitting took to produce an increase in pain was twenty minutes. (You will also see that on one occasion she sat for an hour without any increase of pain – but when you are trying to discover a safe baseline, it makes sense to pick the shortest time recorded; the aim here is to increase your baselines over time, so it pays to be a little cautious at first.) The baseline is calculated as 80 per cent of this minimum figure. The simplest way of working this out is to multiply the time in question by 0.8 – so 20 minutes x 0.8 = 16 minutes. The baseline for sitting in this case is, therefore, sixteen minutes.

In time, you can increase your baseline as your tolerance increases, but you should start at this figure. If you find that your baseline still causes you stress or discomfort, then you should reduce it further and continue doing so until you find one that works for you.

Once you have established your baseline, a timer can help you stick to it. As an example, if sitting causes problems, you could set the timer when you sit down at work, in a meeting or in front of the TV. When the timer goes off, simply move and stretch a little or perhaps lie down for a minute or two. Adapt this approach to suit your condition.

If you want to improve your tolerances – your ability to do a certain task or activity – then you can gradually increase your baselines. You will begin to do this over the coming weeks. Try to remember to be cautious though, and not to fall into a boom-and-bust cycle (see page 119). It is far better to increase your baselines slowly than to overshoot them and crash back to earth.

When working out your baselines, it is best to monitor one activity at a time. Vidyamala began with sitting, as it was obvious from her analysis that this was a particular problem. Discovering the length of time that she could sit without causing a flare-up helped her avoid slipping into another boom-and-bust cycle. Later on, she set baselines for her other activities (see below). In this way, she gradually brought greater balance into her life, slowly improved her overall fitness and reduced her pain, suffering and stress. When you do this yourself, it is

Baseline record example sheet

Baseline record for: SWIMMING

Baseline level: – swim 10 lengths alternating freestyle and backstroke @ 3 times per week. Also do leg exercises at side of pool.

Date	Level achieved	Notes
25th June	10 lengths in morning	Good. Exercises included: 10 each leg backwards and forwards 10 leg lifts 10 leg cross (flared up later, so do less next time)
28th June	10 lengths in morning	Good. Reduced leg exercises to 5 times each leg (still flared up but not as badly).
30th June	10 lengths in morning	Good. Did the same exercises as 28.06 but left out the leg cross exercise (didn't flare up later so will continue this regime for time being).

best to keep a written record of the changes that you make (see Vidyamala's example on the previous page). This is to prevent your state of mind from colouring your memory. You will find a blank sheet for this in the Appendix (see page 259 – and you can also find a template available to download at www.breathworks-mindfulness.org.uk and at franticworld.com).

It's important to develop a Pacing Programme that works for you. These examples are only guidelines, so don't be overly literal or mechanical. It's your life and you will slowly work out what's best for you.

Once you have calculated your baselines, then you can begin. Over the coming weeks, we will ask you to keep an eye on them and to gradually extend them, if that's most appropriate for you.

A word of caution

There will be times over the coming days and weeks when you will find pacing hard to bear. You will often feel that you are failing. This is normal, so don't lose heart. Try to approach it as a long-term project, and with a sense of curiosity and compassion. Living with pain, illness and stress is difficult, and it takes a lot of patience and kindness to bring awareness and dignity back into daily life. Remember, the pacing programme is a tool to help you improve your life – not another stick with which to beat yourself.

It can be hard to pace yourself if you have not, at least to some extent, accepted the reality of your situation. Resistance to pacing is often coupled with a sense of wanting to return to a time when you were completely healthy, pain-free and far less stressed. But in reality, you can either pace yourself – and make the most of your situation – or you can return to the boom-and-bust cycle. Trying to live out a fantasy existence will only lead to sorrow. Eventually, you will have to accept your new reality. This may mean that you'll need to grieve for the mobility, health or energy that you have lost. And while this might sound like a harsh and negative approach, such a compassionate acceptance actually lays the groundwork for making the most of your life. You can then begin to live a life that is more aligned with your condition.

You've started, but must you finish?

'I worked out that I could stand for about ten minutes without an increase in pain,' says Jennie. 'If I'm washing up, I set the timer for ten minutes, and when it goes off I do something else – maybe lying down or sitting down for several minutes. Then I do another ten minutes of washing up. It had never crossed my mind to do that. I had assumed that once you started washing up you carried on until you'd finished. It was revolutionary to think you could stop doing something many times, and then start it again.

'I quickly learned I'd been drawing the wrong conclusions about the increases or decreases in my pain. I knew lying down often made it feel better, so I thought I should lie down for as much time as possible. I also noticed that going for a walk was sometimes beneficial, so I concluded that I should go for long walks. Neither strategy was helpful – I learned that what I needed was frequent changes of activity. A fifteen-minute walk and a ten-minute lie-down were best, and any more lying down produced more pain.

'This immediately gave me a sense of having a choice in dealing with pain, rather than being a victim. I can't control all my external conditions, but I can be more conscious of the choices I make.

'I've learned that to keep my pain within manageable limits: I need to lie down for five minutes every hour and a half; I can't sit at the computer for more than twenty minutes; I can walk for about an hour; I need to do various mindful movements every day; and I can hardly ever sit comfortably in a chair. I've also found, surprisingly, that I can sit in a moving car for three hours, but only for one on a train. The balance of my activities needs to be fine-tuned. For example, in my normal life I need more rest than most people, but on meditation retreats (which I regularly attend), I need to do more activity than everyone else.'

If you have a degenerative disease you may find that your baselines and tolerances decrease over time. It's important to realise this and to make allowances so that you don't feel that you are failing. Richard discovered that he couldn't maintain his baselines over time because of his progressive multiple sclerosis. At first he was despondent, but after a while he began to focus on the practices that he could do and to maintain his baselines as well as he could, making reasonable allowances for decreases over time. This helped him avoid falling back into a boom-and-bust cycle. He continued to attend Breathworks day retreats and drop-in classes for several years as he managed his illness with as much awareness as possible. His gentle acceptance and quiet determination to make the most of his life always had a positive effect on the group.

Sometimes pacing means doing more, not less. We have encouraged you to begin your pacing programme at an easy level. However, you should also bear in mind that you might need to start by extending the amount of time that you spend on your daily activities. Steve discovered this. He has diabetic peripheral neuropathy, which causes pain in his feet. After a few days of pacing, he realised that a daily walk of two hours was far more effective for his pain and blood-sugar levels than a ramble of thirty minutes. So for him, pacing meant that he needed to extend his daily walk, rather than break it up into smaller sections.

Key pacing points

- Remember, pacing is about *taking a break before you need it*. That's the key to maintaining mindfulness and pre-empting the boom-and-bust cycle.

- Start within your baselines, doing only what you're sure you can manage, and gradually increase the amount you do or the time you spend on it. Be ready to leave, for now, those activities that you find too difficult. You can come back to them as you get fitter. Starting with activities that are easier brings confidence.

- By establishing baselines, you will learn to make better judgements about your activities, changes of position and posture and also of rest. Remember to change your position regularly. For example, while preparing a meal, try alternating between standing and sitting, as well as taking a short rest break every now and then.

- Vary the ways in which you use your body throughout the day, making sure that you use different muscle groups. For example, don't try to do all your vacuuming in one day, but spread it over the week. Vary your activities between sitting, walking, standing and lying.

- Keep to your targets and plans as much as you can without being obsessive or rigid. And remember to use a timer.

- On a bad day, try to keep going as planned, but pace yourself more, taking more rest breaks. On a good day, be careful not to do more than you've planned. Avoid overdoing things. This will mean that you, not your pain or illness, will decide how much you do.

- Doing something enjoyable during your rest periods can help you avoid boredom or frustration. Try reading a book or magazine, or listen to the radio or watch the TV.

Following these guidelines, you should have fewer flare-ups, gradually find yourself doing more and regain a sense of initiative and confidence.

HABIT RELEASER: MAKE PEACE WITH GRAVITY

Have you ever spent time thinking about how amazing gravity is? Everything on this earth is held in place by this invisible force that exerts just the right amount of 'pull': too much and we'd be unable to move; too little and we'd float away. We've evolved so that we can function in harmony with gravity. But if you've got difficulties in your life that cause discomfort in your body, you've probably got very deep habits of resisting feeling them – subtly pulling away from the body and, in doing so, also fighting gravity. Every time you pull away from your body in an attempt to avoid feeling it, you're unconsciously creating more suffering, strain and exhaustion. It only makes your pain or stress worse.

The Habit Releaser this week is to let your weight sink *into* gravity with acceptance and self-compassion. Just like in the Compassionate Acceptance meditation practice for this week, allow your awareness to move *towards* your body, to sink into it with kindliness.

This could be when you're driving the car, standing in a queue, sitting in an armchair or lying on the bed – or any other time. Notice if you're subtly pulling away – straining to avoid your experience – and soften into it instead. Give all your weight to gravity and let your whole body feel held and supported by this invisible force. You don't need to hold on at all – let gravity hold you instead. Trust your heaviness and settle into the moment. Vidyamala has been practising this for many years and it has become second nature to her. Before she learned mindfulness she used always to strain away from her pain and her body, and she realised this was making her pain and tension so much worse. What a relief to live with gravity, rather than fight it.

The poet Rilke describes gravity as being like an ocean current that 'takes hold of even the strongest thing and pulls it towards the heart of the world'. He goes on to ask us 'patiently to trust our heaviness' and ends with the beautiful reminder that:

> *Even a bird has to do that*
> *before he can fly.*

CHAPTER EIGHT

Week Five: The Pleasure of Small Things

The surf crashed on to Brighton beach. Ally sat on the shingle, staring at the setting sun, wind gently ruffling her hair. Her legs ached all over, but it didn't seem to bother her so much today. She picked up her notepad and began to write a list with her favourite pen:

'Beautiful sunset, shiny pebbles on the beach, heather still flowering, glistening pavement, soft grass covered with spider webs, rustling leaves, sunshine on eyelashes, crinkly tissue paper, lying down on soft sheets, the smell of woodsmoke, soft woolly jumper, hugs, fresh bread, dark chocolate, more hugs, clean hair, mugs of tea …'

The list was to remind her of all the positive things that she'd experienced that day. Ally sighed and realised that life was good. After pausing to watch the sunset for a few moments more, she picked up her stick and hobbled across the shingle towards Ship

Street for chips and mushy peas. Eating them, soaking up their tastes, aromas and textures, would complete her 'homework' for the day.

Ally was part-way through her mindfulness course, about where you are now, and was doing something that she would have considered impossible just a few weeks previously: she was enjoying life. Although she was still in pain, it had diminished greatly – mainly because she had eliminated so much Secondary Suffering with her mindfulness practice. Ally was pleased with this, but she was learning something even more important: that an enjoyable and fulfilling life is so much more than the absence of suffering. She was learning to embrace life again. Of course she wanted the remains of her pain to vanish (preferably instantly), but she was discovering that it was possible to find pleasure amid her suffering.

We have all marvelled at those who manage to find happiness and 'meaning' while enduring immense hardship. Over the years, a great many studies have sought to discover how some people manage to do this while others do not. Science is now showing the underlying tendencies in the brain that can make it so hard to enjoy life – and maintain an optimistic state of mind – when you are suffering with chronic pain and illness. But more importantly, it has also become clear how you can begin to appreciate life once again and, in the process, kick-start a virtuous cycle that will further diminish your suffering.

It is a sad truism that we humans are hard-wired to suffer. Some of the world's religions say that 'all life is suffering'. Neuroscientists say that we have a 'negativity bias'. Either way, much of our suffering is a side effect of the instincts that nature has built into us through millions of years of evolution.

In a sense, it is a miracle that early humans endured at all. We do not have the sharp teeth and claws necessary to defend ourselves against predators. Nor can we easily outrun them. We do, however, have great cunning and intelligence. We are extremely good at anticipating and avoiding danger. But this has come at a price because it means we have evolved brain systems that focus by default on negative information – to always look on the bleak side of life. True, we respond to the proverbial 'carrots' and 'sticks' (to seek out rewards and avoid threats), but this process has a powerful inbuilt bias. It means our attention inevitably focuses on threats. This is because if you miss a 'carrot' today – a pleasant experience, say – you'll probably get another chance tomorrow; whereas if you fail to spot the 'stick', you'll die and won't get another chance tomorrow. So the compulsion is always to spot the sticks and avoid them at all costs, even if it means that you frequently miss the opportunity of a carrot. Our inherent bias towards negative thinking ensures that we tend to see threats everywhere and notice the flaws in everything. This is the main reason why the mind focuses on pain and suffering with laser sharpness. But far more importantly, it means we simply do not notice the overwhelming number of pleasant things in our lives.

This so-called 'negativity bias' in the brain is incredibly powerful and can sweep all before it. Neuroscientists estimate that it can take as little as a tenth of a second to notice a threat – an aggressive-looking face, for example – and many times longer to notice something pleasant. This is compounded by the fact that threats are reacted to virtually instantaneously and go straight into memory, where they are held on a hair-trigger ready for instant recall, while positive experiences take far longer to sink in. This is why we tend to learn faster from pain than from pleasure. The old saying 'one bitten, twice shy' describes this phenomenon perfectly. In fact, it's estimated that it can take five pleasant experiences to balance a single negative one of equal magnitude.

The neuropsychologist Dr Rick Hanson describes the brain as possessing 'Velcro for negative experiences and Teflon for good ones'.[1] This bias is built into the very structure of the brain and drives all of our instincts and emotions. For example, the amygdala, central to the brain's alarm system, dedicates two-thirds of its neurons to processing negative experiences. And if you should look at brain activity in a scanner, negative experiences generate intense activity, while pleasant ones of equal magnitude produce far less. This bias is reflected in the body's hormonal systems too. We have numerous stress hormones that force us to respond to negative experiences: cortisol, adrenaline and norepinephrine are all fast-acting and have powerful effects on the body. The equivalent 'positive' ones – such as the 'cuddle hormone' oxytocin – lack the same potency and urgency (although they do have powerful effects in the longer run, enhancing health, healing and overall wellbeing).

Manipulated by the negativity bias

'When I learned about the negativity bias,' says Roger, 'everything fell into place. If your fridge breaks down you conclude that "They don't make them like they used to"; when you notice the one bad-mannered person in a crowd you conclude that "The country is going to the dogs". The bias feeds into every toxic state of mind.

'It also explains why the media is dominated by violence and negative news. Those who run the media know precisely how to manipulate us. They frighten us and then offer us shelter. They create a form of instability and dependence in our minds. We watch, glued to the television, as other people suffer, hoping it won't happen to us, before accepting the refuge offered by the advert breaks. All we have to do is buy something we don't want or need and then we'll feel happy and safe. It's a system that works brilliantly for selling us more stuff – and for maintaining social hierarchies – but it also drives mental and physical pain and suffering.

'This used to make me angry – which is another toxic state of mind, of course – but now I simply acknowledge that it is happening. I make sure I press the mute button during the ads. That acknowledgement and simple action means that I'm free once again.'

In short, evolution has given us a brain that routinely tricks us into overestimating threats and underestimating rewards and opportunities. And while this makes evolutionary sense, it can make for a truly miserable existence. But then again, as far as nature is concerned, it is far more important that we survive than be happy.

The negativity bias is also fundamental to our perception of pain and suffering: intense pain and suffering tend to be felt all over the body, while pleasure is normally localised. And, as you will recall from previous chapters, mental anguish drives physical pain and suffering in an endless vicious cycle.

All this may seem a bit, well, negative and hopeless. However, we are not condemned to a life of mental and physical suffering – because the negativity bias can be overcome, and it is to this that we turn this week: it is time to redress the balance. It is time to start enjoying life once again.

Practices for Week Five

- Ten minutes of Body Scan meditation (see page 63; track 1 on the CD), to be carried out on six days out of the next seven.
- Ten minutes of the Treasure of Pleasure meditation (see page 164; track 5 on the CD), to be carried out on six days out of the next seven (ideally at a different time of day from the Body Scan). You can also do extra meditations, such as the Breathing Anchor, immediately before the Treasure of Pleasure meditation to help settle the mind.
- Continue implementing your 'baselines' (see pages 170–4).
- A Habit Releaser: write down ten good things (see page 175).

REWIRING YOUR OWN BRAIN

Understanding the negativity bias is the first step towards rebalancing it. The next is to gently soothe those brain networks that maintain the bias and that, ultimately, lead to unnecessary pain and suffering. As these networks begin to calm down, you can then begin strengthening the brain circuits that notice and appreciate life's pleasures. This rebalancing will help you to see more clearly, act more effectively and be less distracted and rattled by day-to-day life. It will also create a sense of open-hearted calm; the warm and tingling love of life that you probably experienced when you were far younger. As this sense of calm tranquillity builds, it will further reduce your pain and suffering, while dissolving feelings of anxiety, stress, unhappiness and exhaustion.

Rebalancing is achieved by bringing mindful awareness to the small pleasures of everyday life. To do this, we ask you to carry out the Treasure of Pleasure meditation and try, the best you can, to also transfer this quality of open-hearted awareness to the rest of your day. Throughout the next week, bear in mind that it can take a while for pleasure to become rooted in the mind. So try to focus your awareness on the pleasant experience for as long as you can. It can also help to switch awareness between different aspects of the same experience. If you are focusing on eating, for example, instead of solely concentrating on the taste, try soaking up all of the different flavours, aromas and textures as well. Try also to embody what you experience: make a mental note of it, really take it all in, consciously encourage the experience to become a part of you.

This may all seem a little 'woolly', but it is grounded in solid neuroscience. The Canadian psychologist Donald Hebb said: 'Neurons that fire together wire together.' So by focusing on pleasure, you are encouraging the parts of your brain that notice and create the sensations of happiness and pleasure to grow and become stronger – to 'wire together'. This is evidenced by one of the great discoveries of recent years – that the brain is highly 'plastic', which means that it is constantly adapting and changing its architecture. We're not stuck with the brain that we've got: we can change it for the better with mindfulness. Another psychologist, Paul Gilbert, states that we produce new brain cells every day (possibly up to 5,000) in a process called 'neurogenesis'.[2] This shows once again how active and adaptable the human brain is. So if the brain is constantly adapting and changing, we might as well encourage it to move in the best direction. For this reason, mindfulness has been likened to performing surgery on your own brain.

You may wonder why last week you needed to learn how to soften towards your pain before turning towards pleasure this week. Couldn't you just go for pleasure while blocking out the pain? This is an appealing idea, but when you resist and block unpleasant experiences, you also exclude a whole band of sensitivity that includes your ability to appreciate the pleasant, positive and beautiful things in life. Have you noticed how, for example, when you're blocking out pain you find it hard to feel much emotion when you see a beautiful sunset? Or maybe you can't feel much in response to beautiful music? Or maybe it's difficult to be open and receptive to a loved one? It's as if you have become a little brittle – only partially alive – which does not make for a very satisfying and rewarding quality of life. It's important, therefore, first to soften resistance to your pain and become more sensitive and receptive, before fully opening up to beauty and love. And this is an important aspect of mindfulness practice: becoming fully alive and awake to all experiences.

It is a good idea to carry out the meditation while listening to the audio track. By this stage in the programme you may also feel ready to experiment meditating without guidance. By all means try this. Just use the recording for the first few days to become familiar with the meditation. You might also like to extend each meditation by sitting or lying quietly for a short while after the track has finished.

Treasure of Pleasure meditation

This meditation will help you reconnect with the pleasant aspects of daily life.

Preparation

Establish a comfortable meditation posture in the usual way – either sitting, lying or any other posture that will enable you to be as comfortable as possible throughout the meditation.

Gently settle into gravity, allowing your body to be drawn towards the floor, the bed or the chair by the natural force of gravity within which you are resting. Feel your body resting down towards the floor over and over again.

The meditation

As you rest with gravity, very gradually allow your awareness to gather around the movement and sensations of the breath in the whole body. Allow the whole body to be rocked and cradled by the natural breath as it expands on the in-breath and subsides on the out-breath.

Make sure you are open to all of your experience as much as possible – mentally, emotionally and physically – checking in particular for resistance. Are there aspects of your experience that you're pushing away or hardening against? If this is the case, then notice this with acceptance and kindliness and then, very gradually, include these elements within your awareness with a broad and open quality, letting everything be rocked and cradled by a kindly, gentle breath.

And now, on the basis of being awake to all of your experience with this gentle, inclusive, receptive awareness, begin to pay attention in particular to anything pleasant or enjoyable, keeping your focus grounded in the body and the senses. What do you discover? Maybe you notice that your hands are soft and that this is pleasant. Maybe your belly is soft and this is pleasant. Maybe your face is soft and this is pleasant. Bring a gentle, kindly curiosity to your awareness as you learn to pay attention to subtle and quiet experiences as well as strong ones. You may think there's nothing pleasant in your experience at first glance, but as you drop deeper into your awareness and become attuned to more delicate experiences, you may discover that you have more pleasant dimensions to your overall experience than you had previously realised.

Maybe there's even an emotionally pleasant sense of relief as you learn to live with whatever you experience with kindness and acceptance, rather than being trapped in a state of longing for your experience to be different. Your experience is what it is in each moment, and it can be a relief to soften into this, and not struggle and fight against it – being locked into a battle with life.

And what about sounds? Maybe there's a pleasant or enjoyable sound inside or outside the room. Or maybe you're in a very quiet place and that's pleasant. Let the sounds come towards you and include them in your present-moment experience. If you're noticing pleasant sounds, take care that your awareness doesn't fly out the window towards the sound, but rather allow the sounds to arrive in your hearing, in your body.

So spend time resting in a broad and open awareness, allowing anything that is pleasant to rise and fall – enjoying it, appreciating it, resting within it, while staying open to its fluid, changing nature.

If you find it difficult to find anything pleasant, there's no need to worry or judge yourself, just see if you can cultivate a kind, accepting awareness towards whatever your experience is. It's important to remember we're learning how to seek out subtle experience in this meditation practice, rather than noticing only very loud or dominant experiences. The pleasant experiences that you become attuned to may even seem rather ordinary, such as an absence of hunger or a tiny tingling somewhere in your body. But it's important to learn to recognise these, to appreciate and enjoy them.

What's happening now? Are you still finding pleasant dimensions of the moment to rest upon? And if you find your mind is wandering then remember that this is normal. This is what minds do. But each moment you become aware that you've wandered is a moment of being awake, a magic moment. Cherish these moments of waking up from wandering when they occur, and then gently re-engage with the practice of seeking out the treasure of pleasure.

Conclusion

Now broaden your awareness to include the weight of the body, the shape of the body, the breath in the body, sounds and smells. Gradually begin to move the body a little bit and open the eyes. See if you can take this appreciative awareness of the pleasant, even beautiful, with you as you gradually and gently re-engage with your daily activities. Be careful to take time over the transition from meditation to activity – perhaps sitting quietly for a few more moments absorbing your experience.

BRAIN SURGERY

A common initial reaction to this week's practices is a nagging worry that you will find nothing pleasant to focus upon. While this is an understandable fear, truth is, there will always be something pleasant in your life. It might be the sound of a loved one's voice, your favourite food, a long-forgotten piece of music, the smell of freshly mown grass, the feel of sun on your skin or the sound of wind in the trees. We have not yet met anyone who could not find something pleasant when they have consciously sought it out.

The poet Maitreyabandhu captures this beautifully when he says:

There's no law against my listening
to this thrush behind the barn,
the song so loud it echoes like a bell,
then it's further off beyond the lawn.
Whatever else there is, there's this as well.[3]

Craig was a sceptic: 'I was in great pain in hospital a few years ago and was stumped when I was asked by the mindfulness teacher to focus on the pleasant. "What?" I thought. "But I'm in hospital!" I was in pain and there's nothing pleasant about being in an orthopaedic ward after a motorbike accident.

'I gave it a try anyway. I scanned my experience, looking for pleasure, and became aware of how nice it was to lie on clean and crisp sheets. It was surprisingly pleasant. I spent ages just savouring the whole experience. I focused on the textures of the sheets, the way they slid over my skin, and the smell of the cloth. It was lovely to notice these things and to allow them into my awareness. The meditation changed my overall experience, so it became a little less dominated by suffering.'

It can be equally difficult to find pleasure when life in general seems to be conspiring against you. If you are tired, depressed, exhausted or suffering particularly badly, the idea of seeking any form of happiness can seem daunting to say the least. In these circumstances, motivation can be a real problem. This is largely because the 'aims' of the Treasure of Pleasure meditation can seem to be running against the tide of your experience. If you find this to be the case, try remembering that mindfulness has no aims. Instead, it is akin to exploration. You find what you find. Nothing more. You will discover, though, that if you open your mind to the *possibility* of pleasure, you will find it. It appears elusive only because it is obscured by the negativity bias we talked about earlier in the chapter. Pleasure is always there, just waiting to be discovered.

Nevertheless, lack of motivation can be a real problem when life becomes particularly frantic and begins slipping through your fingers. Celine, a ski instructor from Chamonix in France, told us of the time when her eight-month-old daughter woke up at 11.30 pm and refused to go back to sleep until four the next morning. This would be difficult for any parent, but Celine was recovering from a skiing injury that had left her with extremely painful tendonitis in her knees and elbows. To make matters worse, she had recently split up with her partner of six years.

'My daughter was screaming and I could do nothing to calm her down. It was very frustrating and I was exhausted. I tried to relax into these feelings, but mindfulness soon went out of the window. By 2 am I was just a sobbing mess and didn't know how to deal with it. I needed my ex more than ever, but he was off with somebody else.

'The next day my pain levels were alarmingly high and I was very irritable. I thought I'd do a ten-minute meditation to try and calm down. As soon as I lay down to do the Treasure of Pleasure meditation my daughter Amelie wanted my full attention. She began throwing stuff around and tugging at me. This happened just at the point in the meditation track when it says, "Look out for pleasant sensations." I thought to myself, "What? Now? I can't." I thought it was impossible, but then I realised that my pleasant experience could be the sensations of my little girl touching me. So instead of finding her presence irritating, I thought I'd focus on the pleasure it gave me.'

Celine had come to that fork in the road that we all face many times each day. So she decided to try to stop resisting the situation and instead become more accepting of it. She found it very difficult for a while. After all, she was extremely tired and irritable. But then she realised that she was becoming ensnared in Secondary Suffering – and that she could free herself.

'The Primary Suffering was: "I'm tired and in pain." And I couldn't do anything about that. But the Secondary Suffering was my irritation: hating my ex, wanting my little girl to be quiet, wanting to sleep, wanting this, wanting that and wanting just about everything else. After a while I managed to drop the resistance that was stoking my Secondary Suffering. All of a sudden my daughter's little hands felt so sweet as she touched me, rather than being irritating. And I totally relaxed. It was a really drastic change, just from changing my thoughts. In the end, I felt refreshed and the whole day was full of these kinds of little experiences. I'd feel irritated, then manage to identify it as resistance, and then drop the resistance. This process seemed automatically to lead to a pleasant experience and I was very pleased to have turned the day into quite a nice one after all.'

THE PACING PROGRAMME: CONSOLIDATING YOUR BASELINES

Last week we asked you to calculate your baselines. Although your symptoms will vary from day to day, establishing a baseline helps you to set a steady pace that does not exacerbate your difficulties.

This week we ask you to fine-tune your baselines. You will have probably discovered that you are doing some activities for too long while others are easily accomplished. To iron out these inconsistencies, this week we ask you to consciously do two things.

Firstly, those activities that you can do easily, without any flare-up of symptoms, should be carried out at the same level: that is, you should maintain both their duration and intensity. (There will be plenty of time later on to extend them if you choose to do so.) Secondly, those activities that cause a resurgence of symptoms should be carried out for a little less time. Simply do them for about 80 per cent of your current baseline time (see page 147–9 for a quick refresher of how to do this). You can continue reducing your baselines in this manner until you eventually find one that is comfortable. And remember that there is no shame in reducing your baselines. The aim of this exercise is to establish a mindfulness rhythm that is both enjoyable and sustainable, so be prepared to experiment using a light and playful attitude.

The art of pacing is taking a break before you need it. You may find this counter-intuitive because we all tend to do something until it is either completed, or we're forced to stop through pain, exhaustion or stress. However, if you take a break before you are desperate, then you will not only find life more enjoyable, you will end up accomplishing far more too. In a sense, you are learning to conserve your energy, instead of always stretching the limits of your resources. It's a bit like always having some money in the bank or petrol in your car. It gives you some reserves to draw on, rather than running on empty.

Even with the best of intentions, however, it can occasionally be difficult to fit the Pacing Programme into daily life. Allan found this out for himself. He was anxious to get back to work as a geologist for an oil-exploration company. He'd been off sick for three months following a mountain-biking accident and felt that his career was passing him by. Within a day of returning to work, he had a lengthy 'to-do' list and genuinely couldn't find the time for pacing. He discovered that he could slot the daily meditations into his diary, but pacing was another matter entirely. Then it dawned on him that he would never *have* the time. He would have to *make* the time.

'I hate pacing, but I can see that it is very important,' says Allan. 'I find it hugely irritating and I don't want to do it at all. But I'm often confronted with the need to do it when I get to the end of a particularly busy day. It's then that I realise that I haven't made the time to pace myself properly at all and I often feel stressed out and very achy. I've now learned many, many times that I must pace myself. No "ifs", no "buts", I simply have to pace myself.

'I'm slowly learning how to make wise choices about how I prioritise activities throughout my day and ensure I make time to come back to awareness of my body and breath. Sometimes it's just for a few moments, scattered regularly through the day. Other times I make sure I have proper breaks – that's the best way of doing it. These breaks take priority over my work schedule. Yes, it means some things have had to go, but guess what? I don't miss them because I am enjoying my work and my life more. And I'm actually much more productive because I'm not getting so stressed and inefficient. I read once that stress means you can't prioritise any more and that's certainly my experience. I become a bit like a headless chicken if I'm not careful. So overall, I'm making better strategic business decisions because my mind isn't so clouded with pain and I've been able to reduce my painkillers.'

In many ways, the art of pacing is learning to fit it into your life. If you can mindfully take a step backwards, you will frequently find that there are many ways of accomplishing this. Often it can be done in unexpected ways. Frank learned to take breaks when he was pushing his elderly father, who suffers from Alzheimer's, around the park. Every ten minutes he'd stop and say something like, 'Pops, look at the view over there.' This gave him a short break to become more aware of himself and his surroundings. It enabled him to soften his response to his own neck and back pain. In turn, he became more caring and compassionate towards his father, and this helped him to cope with the huge stresses in his own life with a little more equanimity.

Tess learned something similar. She paced herself by taking breaks on successive park benches while she was out walking her dog Tiffin. Instead of rushing, she found that she could appreciate the beauty of the world around her by walking more slowly. As a consequence, she would invariably arrive home feeling far happier and less stressed.

It can sometimes be tempting to become a little 'puritanical' and rigid about pacing. Try not to be. There is no virtue in suffering, in pushing yourself too far or in being obsessive about baselines. Remember they are simply an aid to living with more awareness and freedom, not a stick to beat yourself with. And don't be afraid to use your common sense to try to find other ways to manage your life. If you can find a physical solution to your pain, don't be afraid to use it. Steff, for example, discovered that using a sloping desk at work dramatically reduced her suffering. Likewise, experiment with your environment in the same way as you pace yourself: try different chairs, cushions, mattresses, keyboards, mugs and pans ... the list is endless; try walking, instead of taking the lift (or vice versa); or perhaps try taking the bus or train, rather than driving. Experimentation is the key as it can sometimes be difficult to predict what will relieve your suffering.

As best you can, try to remain mindful while pacing. It will give you unexpected insights that could dramatically reduce your pain. Reina noticed that slouching on the sofa in front of the TV made her pain far worse. It didn't happen immediately – she invariably sat upright at first, but within a few minutes she'd slump to one side. She then realised that sitting in the middle of the sofa was the culprit: this was the softest part and it sagged under her weight. She relieved a lot of her 'evening pain' by sitting on a more supportive part of the sofa. 'It was really that simple,' she says.

Reina also noticed that when she was in pain on the left side of her body, she would be much more tense on that side too. She would then grip things more tightly with her left hand. When she drove she noticed that her left hand gripped the steering wheel like a vice; likewise, when she brushed her hair or lifted a cup of tea or coffee. All of this extra tension made her pain far worse. She also realised that her breathing was often tight, tense and inhibited in daily life – especially when she was in pain. All these things were a revelation. Gradually, bringing awareness into the body and the breath, both in formal meditation practice and in daily life, when combined with pacing, had an enormous effect on her whole life. She's now been practising mindfulness for two years and her pain has largely gone. And when it does come back, she knows what has caused it: she's aware of how stress causes tension in her body and this translates into a 'tightness' around the breath, which then causes further pain. When this begins to happen Reina knows to take some time out, to pace herself with a little more compassion, do a Body Scan, be aware of the breath, be careful about how she moves and to choose her posture more carefully. And when she does all of this, her pain gradually begins to dissolve again.

Dangerous comparisons

Emily has lived with severe pain and headaches since falling face first on to a flight of steps while rushing for a train. She landed on her chin, with the weight of her rucksack adding to the impact. She's struggled with anger and depression ever since. She has also been left with a profound sense of frustration that her pain is getting in the way of the life she craves. Recently, on a Breathworks retreat, she spoke of her journey and how she torments herself by comparing her life with the fantasy perfect one that lies just ahead of her – tantalisingly close, but always out of vision. She has now realised that this constant comparison with not only her own fantasy life, but others' lives, is far more painful than the pain of her injury. She's also learned that when she compared herself with others she always projected perfection on to them, when of course, if she thought about it, they have difficulties in their lives too. The people she compared herself with were also, in her mind, turned into a kind of fantasy amalgam of the qualities of several people, whereas no one is actually like that – no one is that successful and happy or that perfect all of the time. She'd fallen victim to what psychologists call 'upward comparison', coveting a lifestyle that was better than the reality of her own.

Emily began to spend a little time each day focusing on pleasant experiences that were real for her, rather than being so dominated by fantasies and the unpleasant.

Here is one of her lists, written in the spring: 'Iridescent pigeon feathers, being still in middle of busyness, light on York station roof, sunshine through clouds, ploughed fields, first daffodils, looking at photos, lying in a pool of sunlight, hugging family, amazing food, chai tea, candles, weight sinking into floor, light on the wall, colourful cushions, orchid petals, bright yellow roses I just wanted to fall into, seeing friends, smell of wood chips, soft traffic sounds, birdsong.'

Such small but beautiful things can transform your day.

HABIT RELEASER: WRITE DOWN TEN GOOD THINGS

Life can be so full of frantic 'busyness' that it's often hard to notice the good things in life. And often, it is the small things that make us happy: the scent of freshly ground coffee, the sound of a loved one laughing, the feel of clean clothes on the skin. Such tiny, seemingly insignificant things can slip by with barely a ripple.

To remedy this tendency, like Emily in the box above, try noticing the small things in daily life that make you happy. When you become aware of them, simply pause for a while and soak up the pleasure of the experience. Then, at the end of each day, consciously write down at least ten that have made you happy or given you pleasure. They do not have to be grand or dramatic experiences – they might instead include such small things as the sight of sunlight streaming in through a window, the pleasure of talking to a friend, the sound of birds chattering, the feeling of doing a job well or perhaps the simple pleasure of the breath in the body.

It is important to write down ten things and not to stop after you've reached four or five. This is the explicit aim of the exercise – consciously bringing to mind the small, previously unnoticed experiences that would normally slip by and not be remembered. It is also OK to write down some of the same things each day. The aim is simply to take note and remember pleasant experiences, not to compile an exhaustive list. Hold on to this list for a while. You might find it useful later on.

It is said that 'What we dwell on we become', so by dwelling on the pleasant and enjoyable aspects of life, learning to appreciate them and give them your full attention, you will become a person who values the pleasant and loving side of life. Day by day, this will help you to step outside of the battle with pain, illness and stress. You might begin to feel like a tree shedding its old leaves ready for the return of spring.

CHAPTER NINE

Week Six: The Tender Gravity of Kindness[1]

It was a crisp autumn day in the Great Smoky Mountains. A group of Cherokee children had gathered around their grandfather and they were filled with intense curiosity and excitement. A few hours earlier, a fight had broken out between two men and the village elder was called upon to settle the dispute. The children were keen to know what the elder had to say about it.

'Why do people fight?' asked the youngest child.

'Well,' the elder replied. 'We all have two wolves inside us and they constantly do battle with each other.'

'Inside us too?' asked another child.

'Yes, inside us *all,'* he replied. 'There is a white wolf and a grey wolf. The grey wolf is filled with anger, fear, bitterness, envy, jealousy, greed and arrogance. The white wolf is filled with love, peace, hope, courage, humility, compassion and faith. And the two wolves fight constantly.'

'But which wolf wins?' asked another child.

'The one that we feed,' replied the elder.

As you read this now, which wolf are you feeding in your heart? Is it the one that soothes your suffering, the white wolf, or is it the grey wolf that consumes your energy and enhances your pain?

When you are experiencing pain and illness, it is entirely natural to become angry at the injustice meted out to you. Fear can begin eating into your soul. Rosy memories can become tinged with bitterness as you remember the times when you were happier and healthier. You might even become envious of those around you who seem to live more carefree lives. While this is entirely natural, the 'grey wolf' can quickly begin to wreck your quality of life because it is a major driving force behind Secondary Suffering. It is the negativity bias writ large. And while this is regrettable in itself, it also creates far deeper problems because such states of mind can prevent the body from healing. This is because the stress created by the 'grey wolf' dampens the immune system, impairing the body's ability to repair itself. It also prevents the release of the body's natural painkillers, which further heightens suffering.

We are all familiar with the mantra 'survival of the fittest'. So much so, in fact, that we assume it is a 100 per cent accurate view of the world. What is less well known, however, is that 'survival of the kindest'[2] is an equally accurate description of how evolution works. To understand this, it is necessary to think a little deeper about the origins of the brain's negativity bias that we discussed in the previous chapter. This, you will recall, is driven by the need to survive and is, in turn, often best served by being cautious – by avoiding life's 'sticks'. This is the 'avoidance' system. Another aspect of our survival instinct is the drive to seek out new opportunities and resources, life's 'carrots' as it were. This is the 'achievement' system. Both of these driving forces ensured that only the most cunning and adaptable of our ancestors survived. But there is also a third facet to our survival instinct that also governs how we approach the world: it is known as the 'soothing and contentment' system.[3] When we no longer feel the need to constantly defend ourselves against danger, and when resources are abundant, so that we're not struggling merely to survive, we feel a pleasant, bone-deep contentment. We feel 'quiet', soothed, content and peaceful inside. It's a sign that we are happy with the way things are and that we are in tune with our environment. And when we feel safe, we are confident enough to look outwards beyond the immediate needs of survival and are able to live in a more connected and harmonious way with those around us. So we can be kinder to ourselves and to others. This bolsters the social bonds that encourage us to cooperate, rather than compete with each other. And such cooperation was critical for our ancestors because those who were kind and worked cooperatively with each other survived better than those who struggled in conflict and isolation. Hence the phrase 'survival of the kindest'. This soothing and contentment system is of equal importance in the modern world because it helps us achieve a sense of emotional 'balance', to progressively broaden our outlook, and to gain an enhanced sense of perspective. This inner peacefulness and sense of perspective is totally different from the hyped-up experience of many of us in the modern world. It may appear to be 'soft', almost a sign of weakness, but it actually has immense power over the body in the long run because it is intimately connected to health and wellbeing.

The soothing system is largely governed by the 'cuddle' hormone oxytocin and a class of substances known as the endorphins. Oxytocin creates 'luvved-up' feelings of contentment and safety; it is produced by a woman when she gives birth and is released by babies when they are hugged or kissed. Whenever we are touched by another, or feel genuinely loved and needed, oxytocin is released. It creates a feeling of community, belonging, love and safety. This is complemented by endorphins – the body's natural painkillers – which act in a similar manner to opiates such as morphine and codeine. The body is flooded with endorphins after an accident or injury and they are capable of numbing substantial pain; but as well as acting as painkillers, endorphins also create feelings of calm contentment and happiness.

This soothing and contentment system does not just make you feel better, it also improves health and healing. When it is switched on, it is a signal that it is safe for the body to begin focusing its resources on repairing itself. So healing is enhanced. This is in stark contrast to the stress hormones which damp down the immune system and suspend self-repair, so that the body can focus its resources on the immediate needs of survival and either fight or run away from danger.

So the body's soothing system is intimately tied up with kindness, affection and compassion. In turn, such 'white-wolf' emotions encourage the soothing system to release even more oxytocin and endorphins in a positive and self-reinforcing cycle. It is the opposite of the vicious cycles that drive pain and suffering with their associated feelings of anxiety, stress, depression and exhaustion.

It is worth remembering that all three emotional regulation systems are necessary for survival, optimum health and wellbeing.

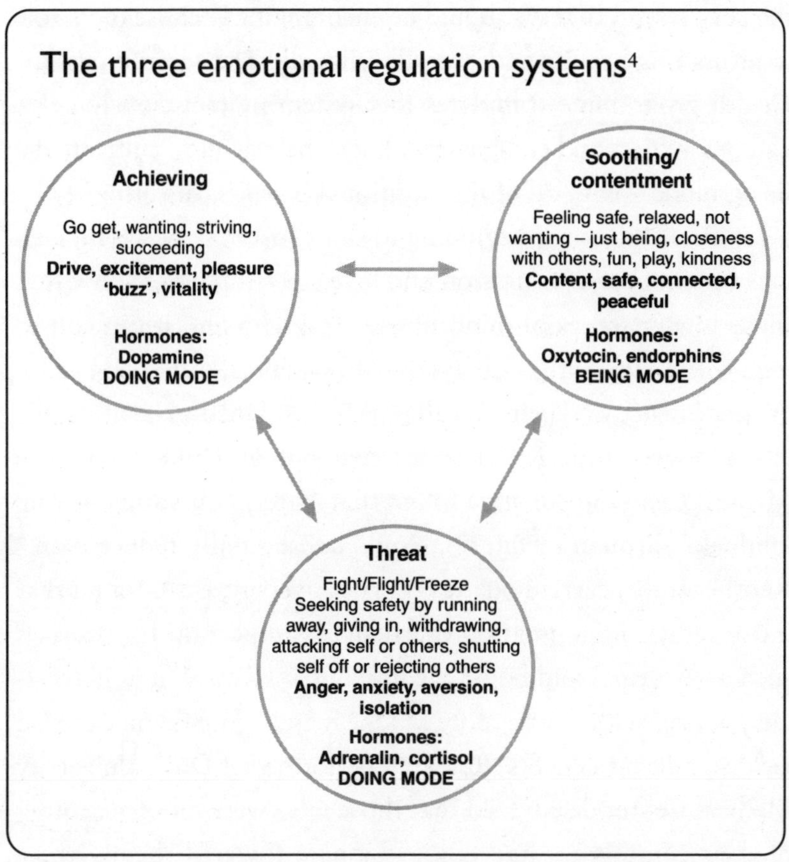

Problems arise only when they drift out of balance with each other, which can happen with chronic pain, illness or prolonged periods of stress. For example, when the threat-avoidance system becomes overactive, we can flail around in fight-or-flight mode, desperately resisting our experiences and becoming increasingly frantic. If the achievement system is overactive, we may drive ourselves brutally hard and seek out distractions as we become increasingly stressed and depressed. Both these systems are the Doing mode writ large. But what this also means is that the soothing and contentment system is underactive – which is, of course, the very system that we should be encouraging because of its role in promoting healing and overall wellbeing. The Mindfulness for Health programme stimulates this system by consciously cultivating kindness and compassion. It also helps you to cultivate the Being mode – with all of the additional benefits this brings.

Clinical studies are beginning to show just how powerful feelings of kindness, compassion and love can be. Studies show that those low in scores of mindfulness, and who find it difficult to treat themselves with compassion and kindness, suffer pain of far greater intensity.[5] Their overall physical and mental health tends to be poorer too. Research carried out at Duke University Medical Center in America found that merely cultivating 'loving kindness' through meditation could substantially reduce pain.[6] Another study, carried out at Emory University, USA, found that it can reduce inflammation (particularly important for diseases such as arthritis) and boost the immune system.[7,8] Simply treating yourself with a little more kindness and compassion can also yield significant benefits. Research performed at Duke University Medical Center discovered that those who were more accepting of their condition – and compassionate towards themselves – suffered far less mental and physical pain. They also found that 'pain disability' – that is the degree to which pain interfered with their life – was far lower than in those who were more accepting.[9] All of this evidence comes on top of the wealth of clinical data that highlights the benefits of mindfulness on general mental and physical health and wellbeing.

Perhaps what is most surprising of all is that these beneficial effects can begin to work after just eight minutes of a specific type of meditation.[10] And it is to this meditation that we will turn to in a moment.

Practices for Week Six

- Ten minutes of the Breathing Anchor meditation (see page 92; track 2 on the CD), to be carried out on six days out of the next seven.
- Ten minutes of the Open Heart meditation (see page 185; track 6 on the CD), to be carried on six days out of the next seven (ideally at a different time of day from the Breathing Anchor meditation). You can also do extra meditations, such as the Body Scan, immediately before the Open Heart meditation to help settle the mind.
- Continue with your 'baselines' (see pages 170–4).
- A Habit Releaser: stopping to look and listen (see page 194).

CULTIVATING A COMPASSIONATE PERSPECTIVE ON LIFE

A central element of this programme so far has been the development of the key mindfulness skill of focusing your mind on a single experience at a time. This is known as 'focused awareness'. It calms and stabilises the mind, thereby reducing anxiety, stress, depression and Secondary Suffering. In Week Four you also learned to bring a sense of self-compassion to your experiences. This 'softening' helped you to accept the changing sensations of pain without automatically adding extra layers of suffering and stress to them. In Week Five you learned to seek out the pleasant and enjoyable aspects of life. This helped you to begin living life to the full once again.

This week you will deepen a second key mindfulness skill known as 'open monitoring'.[11] This is cultivated by observing how your moment-to-moment experience of life constantly changes. It is a theme we have touched on several times before, but this week we will bring it a little closer to centre stage with the Open Heart meditation. This encourages a broad and receptive mind – one that is balanced, stable and non-reactive – and will also deepen your experience of a third and crucial meditation skill, traditionally called 'loving kindness'.

In a sense, weeks Four and Five encouraged you to examine your feelings and sensations of pain and pleasure with great precision and detail, almost as if you were studying them through a powerful microscope. This week we ask you to bring greater perspective into play, to imagine that you are observing your experiences through a wide-angle lens. We ask you to hold on to the full breadth of your awareness, so that you experience everything without becoming embroiled in any one particular aspect of it. A good way of looking at this is to see your mind as becoming a bigger container for your awareness. You will then bring a sense of warmth and compassion to this awareness.

The Open Heart meditation teaches you, deep within your bones, that every aspect of your life is in constant flux. Suffering ebbs and flows. Mountains erode and are washed into the sea. Even the universe – and time itself – will eventually cease to exist. By resting within this sense of oscillation, you will learn to allow pleasant and unpleasant experiences to rise and fall like waves on the sea. In turn, you will no longer feel compelled to habitually grab hold of the pleasant and to resist the unpleasant. And once you can do this, you will be free of suffering's grip.

At this stage, some of these ideas may seem a little too nebulous to grasp, but don't worry – we will guide you through the process step by step. These ideas need to be experienced before you can truly understand them. And that is the central aim of the Open Heart meditation.

The Open Heart meditation

This meditation will help you to cultivate a stable, open, kindly awareness towards all of your experience.

Preparation

As usual, begin by establishing a meditation posture. Align your body as best you can whether you're sitting, lying or standing; and set yourself up to be as comfortable as possible.

Give the weight of your body up to gravity. Allow the whole body to settle down on to the chair, the bed or the floor.

The meditation

Gently rest your awareness inside the body; feel the sensations and the movement of the breath. Can you feel the breath moving inside the body as well as at the edges of the body? Can you allow the front, sides and back of the body to be massaged by the gentle rhythm of the natural breath?

As your awareness begins to settle into the meditation, check that you are not blocking or resisting any unpleasant or painful aspects of your experience. Scan through your body for any feelings of tightness or resistance. See if you can gently and tenderly include these, as well as any pain or discomfort, in your field of awareness with a sense of kindliness. Respond to your pain or discomfort as you'd naturally respond to a loved one who was hurting. Rest here for a few moments and cradle the discomfort in a soft and tender breath. And if you have a strong sense of resistance or aversion to pain or discomfort, or your experience feels hard or defensive, then accept that this is how it is for this moment and cradle *this* in a soft and tender, accepting breath. Allow the weight of the body to settle back down towards the earth with each out-breath, settling over and over again.

Very gently shift the gaze of your awareness to settle upon the pleasant aspects of the moment. Rest your attention, very lightly, on anything pleasant, no matter how subtle: something like the sun falling on your skin perhaps, soft face, warm hands, a pleasant sound or maybe you simply notice an absence of the unpleasant. For example, an absence of hunger. Be careful that you don't only value the big, intense experiences. Remember to pay attention to, and appreciate, the subtle, or even ordinary, pleasant experiences that are always there waiting to be noticed if you include them in the light of awareness in the right way. So gently scan through all of your experiences in the body, in your senses, and rest upon, dwell upon the pleasant and enjoyable.

And now, if you imagine that you've just focused on the unpleasant and pleasant aspects of the moment with a precise and close-up lens of awareness, now very gently broaden and widen your perspective to cultivate a wide-angle lens of awareness. Rest back in your experience, rest back in your body, and allow any unpleasant aspects of your experience to arise and pass away, moment by moment, without resistance or clinging; and allow any pleasant and enjoyable aspects of your experience to rise and fall, moment by moment, without clinging on to them. In the same way as the breath comes into being and passes away, moment by moment, in a continuous flow of movement and changing sensations, allow the unpleasant and pleasant to come into being and pass away in a continuous flow of movement and changing sensations.

If you find images helpful you can imagine that pleasant and unpleasant experiences are like waves on the ocean – continuously rising and falling. If you react to each wave of pleasure or pain with knee-jerk aversion or grasping, your awareness is like a small dinghy or rowing boat bobbing about at the mercy of each wave, each passing sensation. But if you cultivate a broad, stable, non-reactive awareness that includes all of your experience with a sense of wholeness and balance, your awareness becomes like a beautiful streamlined yacht carving its way through the waves and the sea. A yacht has a sense of ballast and depth and also a tall mast providing height and perspective. Can you get a sense of your awareness being like this beautiful yacht as you rest, breathing in and out, including all of your experience within a fluid, open perspective, moment by moment?

Bring a kindly, tender quality to the natural breath. On the in-breath, breathe in kindliness, acceptance towards all of your experience; and on the out-breath, breathe out kindliness and tenderness towards all of your experience.

Rest here for a few moments within this broad, open, stable, kindly awareness towards all of your experience. Instead of your awareness being dominated by the surface waves of the passing sensations of pain and pleasure, see if your awareness can have the perspective of the whole ocean – broad, deep and fluid and saturated with kindness towards yourself. Just as the water of the ocean is saturated with salt, can you let your breath be saturated with kindliness towards yourself?

Conclusion

Very gradually begin to bring the meditation to a close. Form an intention to take this broad and stable, more fluid perspective with you as you move back into your daily life. Allow your body to be grounded, stable and receptive to the kindly breath as you continue to relate to all experience as a flow of passing sensations, thoughts and emotions. Relate to them as they rise and fall, neither automatically pushing away pain, nor clinging on to pleasure.

When you're ready, gradually move your body, taking the kindly breath with you as you move on to the rest of your day.

NEW PERSPECTIVES

It can often be difficult to bring a sense of compassion to yourself and to others. This can be compounded by a struggle to widen the perspective of your thoughts and experiences. The secret is to accept that it *is* difficult. To accept that this difficulty is the way that things *are* for the moment.

Jamie was brutally frank about his struggle with kindness and compassion: 'I felt like a mug, to be honest,' he says.

'I mean, I grew up in Salford. The idea that I could be compassionate just seemed stupid. It seems "weak" and a sign of being a nancy. Let's face it, if you're soft or show any signs of weakness then you'll just be ripped off, won't you? Who should I be compassionate to? The council who doesn't fix my flat? The electricity board? The scumbags outside trying to sell me drugs? Yeah, I had real problems with this week ... I had real problems with this meditation.'

Jamie persisted with the programme, however – not because he wanted to, but because the pain of his crushed left foot forced him to. The first five weeks of the programme had helped him enormously, but after he gave up the course at this point the pain gradually crept back. So after a few weeks he restarted the programme with the Open Heart meditation.

'I just sat and did the meditations. I just wanted to get through this week, that's all. Really, I just wanted to get it over with.'

But then halfway through he realised that he could afford to be compassionate to himself. His mind was his own and nobody need know what was going on inside it, so he could be as kind to himself as he wished. Jamie remained outwardly the same, but inside he was beginning to 'cut himself a little slack', as he put it. After a few more days he grasped what his teacher had been telling him about 'acceptance not being the same as giving up'. It is not passive resignation or indifference. Rather, it is the *active* quality of being fully aware of the real world and of what is happening *around* you and *within* you. This led him to the realisation that his ongoing struggle to be tough was actually weakening him. The constant vigilance and worry had built up immense stress inside him and was preventing his body from healing itself. His foot, crushed by a forklift truck, might never fully recover, but that need not mean that he must live with constant pain.

Anne also realised that her own lack of self-compassion was damaging her health. She had become so wrapped up with her own suffering that life had become intolerably frantic. So she made a strategic decision to embrace the meditation. Her reasoning was that her brain was constantly rewiring itself, adapting to every one of her thoughts and experiences, so she might as well encourage it to move in the right direction.

'I remember the meditation teacher telling us that what you dwell on you become; so little by little, I decided to turn my life around. I wanted to move away from a life oriented around pain and "dis-ease" to one that was infused with a calm tranquillity and a quiet confidence. I wanted to take a step back from my suffering and my struggles so that they no longer bothered me so much. I began by visualising myself as a sleek and stable yacht that slices through the waves of pain and pleasure, rather than feeling like a dinghy being tossed around by the sea. That helped me a lot.

'I won't pretend that it was easy, or that it happened overnight, but it *has* happened. I now feel as if I'm in a calmer place. The pain of my fibromyalgia is now a fraction of what it once was. I just feel so much more in contact with life again. To me, that is priceless.'

Anne learned to take a step back, to listen to the 'white wolf' inside – the voice that's imbued with kindness and compassion. She discovered that if she was to find true peace, then it was necessary to listen to this quiet voice and to ignore the louder ones of fear, anger, guilt and shame. Mindfulness can help us do this, but unless it is imbued with kindness and compassion then it rings hollow. It's almost as if it fails to 'stick' somehow, so you end up dampening down the noise but remain deaf to a better, more wholesome way of living. And it is this better way of living that will dissolve your suffering and help your body to heal.

Megan hit a block at this point in the programme when her illness flared up and she struggled to meditate. Her mind was foggy with medication and she felt nauseous. She'd gained great benefit from the course and wanted to continue, but simply couldn't. Instead of giving up, she found it helpful to think of the course as being akin to a process that spiralled upwards, and not the linear one made up of steady steps that she'd been expecting. Although she was suffering a setback, she realised that she hadn't fallen back altogether – it was more of a process of two steps forwards and one step back. After some initial irritation and disappointment, she began to feel better about the situation. Even though her illness had become especially painful, she knew that she'd become more aware and kind-hearted than she had been at the start of the course. So she stuck with her routine of meditating twice a day, regardless of how she felt during any individual meditation. She understood that the simple discipline of meditating, even if she felt 'all over the place', was still helping to ease her suffering. She also experimented with doing the meditations at different times. She remembered the words of her teacher – that you cannot 'fail' at meditation – and she found this especially helpful when the clouds of doubt and despair drifted into her mind. And every time she noticed that her mind had wandered, she reminded herself that rather than failing she was actually succeeding by experiencing a magic moment of awareness. Gradually her confidence returned and, inch by inch, her suffering began to dissipate once again.

THE PACING PROGRAMME: SETTLING AND BUILDING

At this point in the programme, most people have begun to settle into a regular pacing rhythm. Periods of rest will have begun to punctuate bouts of activity. You may have found that although you appear to be resting more frequently each day, you are also accomplishing more. If you have established such a sustainable rhythm, then you may wish to start extending your baselines. But remember to take baby steps. A reasonable aim is to increase your baselines by a maximum of 5 per cent each week. You can calculate this by dividing your current baseline time by twenty and adding this figure to your baseline. For example, twenty minutes of walking would increase to twenty-one minutes. This does not sound like a lot, but you will be surprised by how quickly you can build up your strength and stamina through regular, paced increases such as this, and it will help you avoid the trap of over-extending yourself and thereby falling back into a boom-and-bust cycle. It's worth bearing in mind that marathon runners avoid burnout by increasing their training intensity by less than 10 per cent each week. So be cautious, and reap the rewards.

If increasing your baselines begins to cause you any undue discomfort, try backing off a little. There is no rush. Remember that this is not an exercise programme: the aim is to help you improve your overall quality of life, so any increase in physical fitness should be seen as a happy side effect.

If you feel that your baselines are sufficient for now, then continue with them for another week. Once again, there is no rush. There will be plenty of opportunities ahead for you to extend them should you wish to do so. Equally, if you feel that your baselines are still too high, then reduce them by about 20 per cent. There is no shame in this. After all, you are still feeling your way forward, so it is perfectly reasonable to spend a little more time experimenting.

CHERISHING THE MOMENTS OF DAILY LIFE

By this stage in the course, many people find that they are also becoming more mindful of daily life in a general sense. You might find that you are stopping more often through the day to appreciate the sun, the sky, the light, awareness of your breath ...

This enhanced awareness crept up on Jill. She noticed it first when she observed tension in her shoulders and chest when she'd been shopping. She gradually learned to drop her shoulders, relax her jaw a little and soften her breath. Then she'd focus on the 'grounded' feelings in her feet. She'd check her thoughts, or see if she was resisting anything, and then soften around that. Each time she caught herself frantically rushing about she would ask herself, 'Why am I rushing?' and check if it was really necessary. Usually it wasn't. Then she would look out for pleasant sensations. These helped her to land in the present moment and remember that life is to be savoured, not rushed. Jill also tried to remember to be particularly mindful of activities that were painful for the tendonitis in her arms – like brushing her teeth and hair or washing her hands. Just taking a little more time over these things made them less painful. She discovered something else too: that taking a little extra time over daily tasks such as these made them more pleasant.

'Who would have thought that the feeling of brushing your teeth could be pleasant?' she told us. 'It felt like my gums were being massaged. I no longer notice the pain from the tendonitis so much. Now I almost look forward to brushing my teeth because I'm doing it more slowly and the whole "getting-it-over-and-done-with" attitude is not there any more – which is really nice.'

Lizzie also learned to delight in daily mindfulness: 'I've begun to live more days that are very mindful. I've allowed a gentleness and spaciousness around everything that I've been involved with, without being driven in the way that I usually am. The low-level anger that lives in me, that is at the back of everything, just doesn't seem to be there any more. I've become nicer to be around and so it's been a good experience for my partner as well. To have a day of kindness to myself, it's nice. It seems as if the more fully I am able to be in my body, moment by moment, then more of me is available to see what's going on in the wider world too. Each time I catch myself speeding up, I know that I am going into automatic pilot, so I consciously slow down again, especially when it comes to how I move around. I know it sounds a bit crazy, but I actually say to myself, "I am walking, I am lifting, I am doing." This is a great way to bring myself back to the present moment. When I sort out my washing, for example, I try to do it really slowly. I feel the texture of the clothes. It's beautiful. The slowing down is key – not pushing through life in my usual hard-driven way. I now have a little mindfulness checklist to carry with me in my wallet. I've stuck a copy on my fridge too. It says: "Slow down. Breathe. Feet on Ground. Breathe. Soften Resistance. Breathe. Enjoy the Moment." I've found this simple thing very helpful indeed.'

HABIT RELEASER: STOPPING TO LOOK AND LISTEN

This week the habit releaser is to stop for five minutes each day to simply look around you or listen to sounds. Adopt a comfortable posture – sitting, lying or standing – and allow experiences to arrive at your senses without telling yourself a story *about* the sights or sounds. Experiment with sounds on one day and with sights on the next, unless you have an impairment, in which case choose the sense that is most vivid for you.

In the case of sounds, see if you can let them come fully to your hearing just as they are – arising and passing away, moment by moment, simply as sounds, as sense impressions. Notice any tendency to try to push away or block out sounds that you don't like. Also notice those sounds that tend to draw you *into* them, so your awareness flies out of your body towards the sounds. You might find yourself trying to work out what they are or perhaps catch yourself making up stories about them and end up in day-dreaming. The practice is to try to be aware of sounds *as* sounds, as changing experiences, while you stay embodied and grounded in broad awareness. Accept the sounds that you don't like and enjoy those that you do. Acknowledge them all and let them go, moment by moment. Notice how they constantly change. You'll probably become restless or bored and feel self-conscious – this is all a normal part of the process. Can you stay open to the boredom, rather than rushing off to do something else?

Do exactly the same thing when you open up to sight. Be open to whatever is within your field of vision. You might like to look out of the window or around your room, or perhaps lie outside looking up at the trees and sky. See if you can have a broad awareness that is open to the various different shapes and colours. Can you let these impressions rise and fall without fixating on any one aspect of them? Be aware of all the different qualities of the sights and of your own mental and emotional processes.

Jean sat experiencing sight impressions in her room in Manchester. It was grey and wet outside, so she decided to look at a print on her wall. She found it fascinating to see how her mind started making up stories about the painting. The first thing that happened was she started remembering the holiday where she'd bought it. Then she noticed how she responded to different elements of the picture and started trying to make them into a story – wondering what the painter had in mind when he painted it. She caught her mind doing that and came back again to 'just looking'. She now found the thinking part of her brain started to let that go at least a little, and she was more able to just look at the various shades of blue and how beautiful they were. She felt more and more drawn into the painting and the beautiful colours. She connected with an inner sense of freedom just from sitting quietly and looking at the painting without the constant chatter of her 'thinking mind'.

Jeremy was fascinated by what happened when he listened to sounds: 'I heard a pneumatic drill in the street outside my room and immediately my mind was out on the street ranting, "Can't you shut up. That's a horrible noise. Why are you drilling, anyway? You're such a useless council. You never fix anything properly." I caught what I was doing and had to laugh at myself! I had created a whole story about the council, when all I knew for certain was that there was the sound of a drill outside – I had no idea who was actually doing the drilling. For all I knew, it might have been the water board repairing the leak I'd complained about. I brought my awareness back into my body again and just let the sounds of the drill come and go, simply as sounds without all these stories. I discovered that there were aspects of the sounds that were quite pleasant. Well, that was a surprise, I can tell you. When the drilling stopped I enjoyed the silence and then the sounds of the birds started to come back and they were pleasant too. But I made sure I let the sounds come towards me in the room, rather than my mind flying off outside.'

CHAPTER TEN

Week Seven: You Are Not Alone

> A human being is part of the whole, called by us 'universe,' a part limited in time and space. We experience ourselves, our thoughts and feelings, as something separate from the rest – a kind of optical delusion of consciousness. This delusion is a kind of prison for us, restricting us to our personal desires and to affection for a few persons nearest to us. Our task must be to free ourselves from this prison by widening our circle of compassion to embrace all living creatures and the whole of nature in its beauty.[1]
>
> ALBERT EINSTEIN

Roseto, Pennsylvania, looks just like any other small American town. Brick and shutterboard houses line the streets; bright red standpipes can be seen on every corner; and overhead traffic lights sway gently in the breeze. It is completely ordinary in every respect, right down to the most common causes of death. But it hasn't always been this way. Until relatively recently, the people of Roseto reported very low levels of stress and had an astonishingly low death rate from heart attacks. It was so low that scientists from across America spent decades studying every aspect of the town to try to establish why Rosetans were so healthy. And their findings highlight the underlying causes of many of the physical and mental-health problems that are sweeping the developed world.

The story begins in 1964 when the *Journal of the American Medical Association* published the results of the first systematic study of mortality in Roseto.[2] Researchers led by Dr Stewart Wolf, head of the Department of Medicine at the University of Oklahoma, discovered that Roseto's heart-attack mortality rate was zero for those under forty-five. It wasn't much higher for men in the 'killing fields' of late middle age. And even for men over sixty-five, it was half the US national average. To make matters even more intriguing, other towns near Roseto had heart-attack death rates that were substantially higher. Further studies ruled out genetic or other physical origins for the Rosetans' good health and general happiness. Nor did they live a conventionally healthy lifestyle. They tended to smoke unfiltered cigars, and both men and women drank wine with seeming abandon. And although the Rosetans were of Italian origin, they had long since substituted lard for healthy olive oil. Even their meatballs and sausages were fried in lard and they ate lots of fatty cheeses and salami. Their jobs could hardly be considered low-stress either. Many worked in the nearby slate quarries, notorious for industrial accidents and toxic dust and fumes. Given all this, the Rosetan mortality rate should have been far higher than the national average, not lower. Two other statistics about Roseto stood out: the crime rate was zero and applications for welfare benefits weren't much higher.

Scientists eventually pinned down the reasons for the 'Roseto Effect' to a strong and caring community made up of close-knit families. Other factors isolated by the researchers included low income disparities, a rejection of ostentatious shows of wealth and the active avoidance of 'consumer culture'. Taken together, these factors were at least as powerful as the normal attributes of a healthy lifestyle such as giving up smoking and regular exercise. At the end of their analysis, the scientists made a prediction: death rates would begin to increase when the residents began to abandon their traditional close-knit culture and to adopt a lifestyle more typical of the developed world.

As the years passed, Roseto progressively moved from being a small, isolated town in rural Pennsylvania to become part of the commuter belt for nearby cities. Some people even began commuting to New York, 75 miles distant. Large houses with high fences were built on the outskirts of town. People began to drive more, and those who could afford to replaced their Fords and Cadillacs with BMWs and Mercedes. In parallel with these changes, the traditional social clubs went into decline and families stopped taking walks together on warm summer evenings. Church attendance – once a central focus of the community's social life – declined. Within a generation, Roseto was transformed – as were the health and wellbeing of those who lived there. So much so that in 1971, for the first time, a person under the age of forty-five died of a heart attack. Roseto's changing tide was documented in 1992 by a study published in the *American Journal of Public Health*.[3] Dr Wolf's original prediction was proven correct: as Rosetans adopted a typical 'individualistic' and highly stressed Western lifestyle, their health and wellbeing declined.

In a sense, the Roseto Effect was entirely foreseeable. As we saw in previous chapters, our instincts encourage us to seek and reciprocate the love and support of our family, friends and community. So when society begins to dissolve, and the invisible web of support weakens, stress levels start to increase and overall health begins to suffer. This process is writ large in much of the developed world, but was largely absent from Roseto until recent decades. And studies around the world have confirmed these findings: people who feel part of society, who believe that their life has inherent purpose and meaning and who freely give and receive help and support from others, tend to be happier and healthier.

While Roseto was clearly a happy and healthy town, it was hardly a Utopia. Life was undoubtedly hard for those working in the slate quarries, the women of the town must have felt frustrated by the paternalistic culture and the young were stymied by the lack of career opportunities. Nevertheless, in health terms at least, these downsides were mitigated by the sense of family and community.

It is clearly fruitless to idolise the past or to try to recreate an idealised version of Roseto. It is sensible, however, to try to recreate the Roseto Effect without also duplicating its downsides. Fortunately, it is possible to do this, even if you live alone or feel isolated from mainstream society. In previous chapters we saw that treating yourself with a little more kindness, compassion and acceptance is good for overall health and wellbeing. You have probably already noticed the benefits (although they can take several weeks to accrue). But the town of Roseto shows us that this is not quite enough. We also need to widen the circle of compassion a little bit further to encompass all of those who share our lives, no matter how fleetingly. And it is to this that we turn this week.

Practices for Week Seven

- Ten minutes of Open Heart meditation (see page 185; track 6 on the CD), to be carried out on six days out of the next seven.
- Ten minutes of Connection meditation (see page 205; track 7 on the CD), to be carried out on six days out of the next seven. You can also do extra Body Scans or Breathing Anchors during the week, or any of the other meditations that seem particularly appropriate to you.
- Pacing with the Three-minute Breathing Space meditation to be carried out at least twice a day (see page 215; track 8 on the CD).
- A Habit Releaser: commit some random acts of kindness (see page 217).

FROM ISOLATION TO CONNECTION . . .

During the programme so far you have primarily cultivated awareness and kindness towards yourself. You have developed the ability to know, moment by moment, what thoughts, feelings and sensations are flowing through your mind and body. In turn, this has helped you to respond to thoughts and sensations, rather than automatically reacting to them. You will have also felt the power of acceptance and compassion first-hand and this, in turn, will have helped you to appreciate life's simple pleasures. Crucially, you have also learned how to saturate your awareness with warmth and kindness, and to begin treating yourself as you would naturally respond to a loved one who was suffering.

This week you are going to take these skills and extend the circle of compassion a little wider to include the other people who share your life – and, ideally, beyond. We are asking to you to put the Roseto Effect into practice. The meditation asks you to develop feelings of love, kindness and social connectedness, and then to extend them ever further outwards. No matter how isolated you might initially feel, this meditation will help you become more complete, grounded and whole.

As with previous weeks, we ask you to do two ten-minute practices a day – preferably the Open Heart meditation in the morning and the Connection one in the afternoon or evening. If you have a little more time, you'll gain great benefit from doing an additional Open Heart meditation immediately before the Connection one. This will allow you to bring kindness to yourself before spreading it outwards to include others. And feel free to experiment with unguided meditation sessions now you are becoming more experienced, if this appeals to you.

A word of warning about the week ahead: when life becomes dominated by problems and suffering, it can be difficult to extend warmth and compassion to others. Pain and suffering can make you feel extremely isolated. This is yet another symptom of stress. And over the months and years, this symptom can become progressively more *real* as physical pain can indeed isolate you. That is why this week's Habit Releaser encourages you to take concrete steps to begin reversing this trend by committing random acts of kindness for another person (see page 217). Nevertheless, if you *are* isolated and feeling chronically lonely, then you might find the Connection meditation a little daunting at first. If this is the case for you, then as best you can, just take baby steps forward. There is no rush. And, as always, try to remember that you cannot 'fail' at meditation. No one is keeping score and you shouldn't do so either. No one is expecting you to suddenly start loving the world and everyone in it. Rather, we ask you to simply follow the instructions as far as possible. Rest in the knowledge that a pleasant side effect of the meditation is that it will slowly but surely help you to become less lonely. A good way of looking at this process is to imagine that you are waking up from a long slumber. You would not suddenly leap out of bed, but would instead gingerly step on to the floor before very slowly lifting yourself upwards. You should take a similar approach to this meditation. It is enough to incline the mind in the general direction of warmth and compassion for others. This will slowly move the tectonic plates of the mind towards kindness and openness. It is a powerful meditation that will, over time, transform your life.

Dr Barbara Fredrickson from the University of North Carolina at Chapel Hill has spent many years studying loving-kindness-based meditations, of which the Connection is one. Her team's research has discovered that they are particularly powerful at defusing the symptoms of chronic pain and suffering.[4] She describes the process thus: 'When people open their hearts to positive emotions, they seed their own growth in ways that transform them for the better.'

With the Connection meditation, more than any other, it pays to remember that perfection is impossible. The only thing that is important is that you simply try, as best you can, to extend your warm thoughts and feelings to others, while contemplating all that you have in common with them. More than this, you cannot do.

The Connection meditation

This meditation encourages you to develop feelings of love, kindness and social connectedness.

Preparation

Establish your meditation posture. Position your body so you will be as comfortable as possible, yet relaxed and alert, for the next ten minutes. Let your body settle down towards the chair, bed or floor, allowing gravity to support your whole body.

The meditation

Rest your awareness inside the movements and sensations of the breath in the whole body – feeling the breath in the front, the back and the sides, the insides of the body and the surface of the body. Allow the breath to be saturated with kindliness and tenderness towards yourself. Saturate your breath with kindliness the way the water of the ocean is saturated with salt. Can you allow all the unpleasant and pleasant aspects of your experience to arise and pass away in each moment within a broad and open field of awareness? Neither pushing away the unpleasant nor clinging on to the pleasant, but resting back within a broad, stable, kindly field of awareness that contains everything with a quality of fluidity and receptivity.

And now bring to mind a friend. Someone for whom you have existing feelings of liking or friendliness. Choose someone as a representative of all the people you like in your life. Now imagine inviting them into your field of awareness, either as an image, a feeling or any other imaginative way that works for you. Stay grounded in your own experience and expand your awareness to include your friend. Sit quietly with them in your imagination, gently breathing together. And reflecting on all that you share with your friend. Although you look different and the details of your lives are different, you're both breathing in and out in exactly the same way, and beneath relatively superficial differences you are so alike. Your friends will have unpleasant experiences they tend to resist and push away or get overwhelmed by and pleasant experiences they tend to cling on to, in pretty much the same way as you do. So see if you can imaginatively reach over the sense of difference and separation that we usually feel towards others and focus instead on a sense of common humanity with your friend. Include a sense of kindliness in the breath towards your friend. On the in-breath breathe in as strong a sense of connection with your friend as you can manage; and on the out-breath breathe out kindliness and well-wishing towards your friend. Everything that you wish for yourself – compassion, contentment, fulfilment, perhaps – you can now wish for your friend. Imagine them being bathed in these qualities with each out-breath.

And now broaden your awareness still further to include other people. Expand your awareness so it radiates out from the centre of your body to include yourself and your friend, and bring to mind other people in your vicinity. Maybe there are others in the house with you or in the neighbourhood. Bring these people to life in your imagination. Each one of them is a living, breathing human being just like yourself. Everything that you experience in your own life, they experience in their lives in their own way. They're breathing in and out every moment just like you. They have unpleasant experiences that they dislike and push away or get overwhelmed by just like you, and pleasant, enjoyable experiences that they can delight in, but so often destroy through grasping – just like you. Spend a few moments feeling a sense of commonality with all these other people.

Now broaden out your awareness still further to include more and more people. See if you can use your self-awareness as a touchstone for empathy with humanity. Instead of feeling isolated by your experience, can you empathise with other human beings as you realise how alike we all are deep down? To the extent that we know ourselves, honestly and authentically, we know humanity. To the extent that we acknowledge our own suffering, we know what it's like for others to suffer. To the extent that we know our own openness of heart, joy and happiness, we know what it's like for others to have joy and happiness and we can delight in this.

And now include kindliness and well-wishing with the breath as you reflect on all that you share with others. On the in-breath, breathe in empathy for all humanity, and on the out-breath, breathe out kindliness and well-wishing towards all humanity. Instead of focusing on difference, focus on commonality. Instead of focusing on isolation, focus on connectedness. Breathe in a sense of interest and connection with humanity and breathe out kindliness and well-wishing to all humanity.

And allow your breath of well-wishing to flow equally towards everybody without preference: people you like, people you don't like; people you know, people you don't know; people who are awake, people who are asleep; people who are nearby, people who are far away; people living in peaceful places and people living in war zones. They're all human beings. We are all so similar. None of us likes to suffer and we all want to be happy.

Rest back within a broad and open field of awareness, remaining centred and grounded in your own experience and expanding your awareness on and on and on to include all life everywhere. Rest inside the movements and sensations of the breath in your own body and have a sense of the whole world breathing – expanding and subsiding, expanding and subsiding. A ceaseless, gentle movement and flow. Allow the whole world to be bathed and saturated in a kindly, loving breath – in and out.

Conclusion

Now very gently, begin to bring the meditation to a close. Maintain a sense of openness towards yourself and towards others with a sense of softness in your body and the breath. Gently open your eyes and move your body, seeing if you can take this quality of connectedness with common humanity with you as you re-engage with the activities of your day. Take time as you make the transition from the meditation space to your daily life.

COMING HOME TO WHO YOU ARE

One of the most common concerns raised about the Connection meditation is that it might make you overly 'soft' or 'weak'. If you have spent months and years struggling with pain, illness or stress, then you will have built protective walls around yourself. Just getting through the day can require a supreme effort of will. After all, you have to be tough, don't you?

While this has an element of truth to it, it's not the whole story. You do need a degree of fortitude to cope with suffering, and mindfulness certainly helps with this, but it also helps you to cope with life's difficulties more skilfully.

Joe had these concerns throughout the course and his worries came to a head with the Connection meditation. He could see the point of treating himself with a little more kindness and compassion, but baulked at offering it to others. The idea of developing even-mindedness was particularly unsettling. 'Isn't that a bit bland and insipid?' he asked. Joe was passionate about life and was worried that this meditation might make him a bit too calm and, frankly, dull. He knew that being reactive, rather than responsive, wasn't ideal, and that constantly feeling on the back foot did make his pain and stress worse – but at least that way he felt alive. Nevertheless, he persevered with his practice. After a while he realised that he could hold both the pain and the pleasure in his mind at the same time. This tempered his pain somewhat. He also saw that there was an element of joy lying just beneath the surface. As his stress began to dissipate, he started to see other people as fellow travellers through life, rather than as hostile opponents needing to be outwitted. This shift in perspective further lessened his stress and suffering. As the benefits took root, Joe volunteered to work in a charity shop that helped the homeless. He didn't want to. In fact, he initially hated the very idea, but he decided to follow the advice of his mindfulness teacher and become more involved with his community. He approached the voluntary work with as much warmth and open-mindedness as he could muster. He remembered the words of his teacher: 'It is enough to incline the mind towards warmth and compassion for others. The rest will follow.'

When he did this, Joe found it a revelation that he could be open to everyone he met, rather than trying to avoid or judge them, based on some initial superficial impression: 'Sometimes it was simply that I didn't like the clothes they wore,' he said. 'That can obviously be a major issue when you work in a shop with a lot of people passing through. After a few days of thinking such thoughts, I realised how petty and small-minded it made me. It was difficult, but I did open up – even if only by millimetres at a time.'

'In a funny kind of way, I needed to be given "permission" to treat others with a little more kindness and respect,' he says. 'That's what the mindfulness course gave me. I would never have thought of taking part in the community before the course. It just wasn't what I was about. Being encouraged to do so meant that I gave it a go. It has made such a big difference to me. I no longer feel so alone. It has brought me out of myself enough for me to never want to go back to my old self again.'

Lisa's story is similar to Joe's, but she felt even more chronically overwhelmed and bullied by the pain of her lupus and the accompanying feelings of isolation. These had led to a growing sense of cynicism in her heart. She could just about bring herself to show kindness and compassion towards herself, but struggled with extending it to others. Lisa eventually opened up to the quiet, soothing voice inside. But she had spent so many years feeling isolated and fearful that it was difficult. Very difficult. She gradually learned that the dominant voices – those of fear and guilt – were drowning out the softer ones of warmth and friendship. She learned what countless others before her had found – that to find true peace it is necessary to listen to the quiet voice of compassion, and not the bellowing ones of fear and anger. Meditation can help us do this, but it is necessary to imbue it with warmth and compassion for others. Otherwise, we run the risk of finding temporary respite and not true peace. Many studies have now confirmed this. Imbuing mindfulness with kindness and compassion switches off the brain circuits responsible for creating tension and stress. And this ultimately damps down pain and suffering. This is what Lisa found out for herself. As her feelings of fear and isolation melted away, she began to feel less stressed, more complete and in considerably less pain.

Belinda also worried about this meditation. She feared that focusing on herself – and then extending this to others – might make her feel even more lonely. Isolation was a deep-seated source of pain for her. She had spent several years suffering from chronic fatigue syndrome following chemotherapy for cancer. After being discharged from hospital, she'd spent several months largely confined to her bedroom, with carers coming in to help her. She was young, intelligent and previously full of life, so she found this situation extremely difficult. She felt trapped by her suffering.

The benefits of connecting with others through the mind came as a revelation to Belinda. At the end of each meditation session, she was still the same woman, in the same physically isolated situation, and yet she felt her mind and heart were transformed.

She realised that in the past, her feelings of envy and of being 'different' had been isolating her from the world. This changed when she began to feel the connections she shared with others. She found it helpful to think of everybody else as breathing just like her; as having the same basic desires to be happy and to avoid unhappiness; as well as the simple fact that everybody else also suffers, not just her. This made her feel more open and compassionate towards the few people she came into contact with. But, more importantly for her, she began to feel less alone too.

One evening she lay on her bed and looked out of the window. She could see houses across the valley and watched all the lights twinkling inside the windows. As she did so, she thought of all those people breathing; all those people living their lives that were not so different from hers. She felt the breath in her own body as if it was at the core of everyone's being. She suddenly felt part of the world. It was a radically new perspective for her.

Iain found that the Connection meditation altered his dealings with those around him in subtle and unexpected ways. Initially, he didn't realise it was having any benefits at all. But then he noticed that he felt much more open and kindly towards a woman serving him at the supermarket checkout. Then, as he walked down the street, he suddenly saw other people as human beings just like him – and then he realised how often he related to other people as objects. This was a bit of a shock. He'd never really thought about how he viewed others, but he saw now that they could have been a tree or a car for all the care that he'd felt for them. Now he saw them in a new light: as human beings just like him – the centre of their own web of relationships, hopes and fears, sufferings and joys. As this realisation slowly dawned on him, Iain began to feel more connected and caring towards them. He found himself smiling as he walked down the road with this new sense of connection with others. Over the next few days, he began to feel the tendrils of stress uncoiling, and with them his pain began to ease further.

THE PACING PROGRAMME: THE THREE-MINUTE BREATHING SPACE

You have probably become increasingly sensitive to the impact that your patterns of rest and activity have on your levels of pain, stress and fatigue. If you have not yet found a comfortable balance, then continue to experiment with your baselines this week to find a pattern that suits you. There is no rush. Finding and adjusting your baselines should be seen as a work in progress, rather than as a definite goal.

If you have found a comfortable balance, then consider increasing your baselines slightly. Always try to remember that there is no rush. Simply move forwards at a pace that suits you. It's also worth bearing in mind that you should not increase any of your baselines by more than 5 per cent each week.

Have you noticed a nagging desire to abandon the Pacing Programme and carry on with your life regardless? When you are feeling happy, pain-free and energised, it can be difficult to remember why you should stick to your baselines. And the opposite is also true: when you feel overwhelmed with pain, stress or anxiety, then motivation can be a huge problem. This is hardly surprising. After all, when you are in pain, you just want it to stop. When you are unhappy, you just want it to go away. And when you are stressed or angry, it's difficult to remember why you should remain calm. In times such as these, mindful awareness tends to evaporate, and the last thing you want to be is mindful. So it's no surprise that tired, old habits can rear their heads. The Three-minute Breathing Space was created for just such times as these. It is a 'mini-meditation' that serves as a bridge between the longer and more formal meditations and the demands of everyday life. It allows you to regularly 'check in' with yourself and to observe unpleasant thoughts and sensations as they arise and then pass away again. In this way, it helps you regain a sense of being 'grounded' with warmth, kindness and safety. Many people say that it's one of the most important skills they learn on their mindfulness course.

The meditation has three main benefits. Firstly, it serves as a means of punctuating your day, so that it's easier to maintain your Pacing Programme. Secondly, it helps to defuse negative states of mind before they can gather unstoppable momentum. (If left to themselves, these may spiral out of control and enhance Secondary Suffering.) Thirdly, it's an emergency meditation that you can carry out in times of acute crisis or pain to soothe your suffering.

The meditation is composed of three stages of roughly one minute each. In effect, it condenses the main elements of the whole mindfulness programme into three minutes. A good way of viewing it is to imagine your awareness moving through an hourglass shape as the meditation progresses. At first, we ask you to become fully aware of the thoughts flowing through your mind and the sensations in your body in quite a broad sense. We then ask you to gather up and focus your awareness on the sensations of the breath as it flows into and out of your body. And finally, we ask you to expand your attention outwards again, to encompass your whole body and to imbue what you find with warmth and compassion. You then expand your awareness even further to re-engage with the world.

The meditation should be carried out at least twice each day, but preferably three or more times.

The beauty of the Breathing Space meditation is that it can be performed virtually anywhere. It works equally well at work, at home, in queues or on trains, the Tube or buses. Nor does it need to be confined to your Pacing Programme. Whenever you feel overwhelmed, the Breathing Space is waiting.

Three-minute Breathing Space meditation[5]

Step 1: arriving

Become still wherever you are – either lying, sitting or standing, choose a posture where you'll be as comfortable as possible, then lightly close your eyes. Bring your awareness to whatever is going on for you right now.

Give the weight of your body up to gravity. Allow your weight to sink into the points of contact between your body and the floor, chair or bed, whether that's your feet, your buttocks or your back.

- What *sensations* are there, right now? If you notice any tension or resistance towards painful or unpleasant sensations, gently turn towards them. Accept them as best you can. If you begin to tense around the breath, then let go a little bit with each out-breath. Soften into gravity.

- Notice any *thoughts* as they arise and pass away in the mind. See if you can let them come and go without becoming too identified with their content. Look 'at' your thoughts, not 'from' them. Observe them as if they were clouds in the sky. Relate to them as a flow of mental events. Remember: 'thoughts are not facts'.
- Notice any *feelings* and *emotions* as they arise. Can you let these come and go without pushing away those that you don't like, or jumping on to those that you do like? Include everything within your awareness with a kindly perspective.

Step 2: gathering

Allow your awareness to gather around the experience of the breath in the body. Drop your awareness inside the breath and feel the different sensations in the front, back and sides of the torso, inside the torso and on the surface of the torso. Feel all of the different sensations of the breath as it flows into and out of the body. Can you rest within the flow of the breath? Let everything change, moment by moment. Use the breath to anchor your awareness in the present moment and the body. Each time you notice your mind has wandered, remember that you are having a 'magic moment' of awareness. You have 'woken up'. Then gently bring the mind back to the breath deep in the body.

Step 3: expanding

Gently broaden and expand your awareness to include the whole body. Feel the weight and shape of the body as it sits, stands or lies.

Feel the breath in the whole body. Imagine you are breathing in and out in all directions: 360-degree breathing. If you have any pain or discomfort, make sure your awareness stays open to include this with a sense of compassion. Soften tension and resistance with each breath. Cultivate acceptance for all of your experience. Befriend it. Now broaden your awareness even further to become aware of sounds both inside and outside of the room. Be aware of other people around you. Then imagine expanding all of your awareness outwards to include all humanity. Imagine the whole world breathing.

Now gently open your eyes and move the body. As you re-engage with the activities of your day, see if you can carry the awareness that you've cultivated with you.

HABIT RELEASER: COMMIT SOME RANDOM ACTS OF KINDNESS

One of the most magical ways of improving another person's life is to commit an unexpected act of kindness. So each day this week, carry out a small good-natured deed for someone else. If you are feeling especially bold, you could be kind to someone you normally find difficult or even dislike. Try to remember that the joy is in the giving, rather than in the gratitude you'll receive in return. You needn't give big presents or make extravagant gestures. Holding open a door or buying a friend or colleague a drink counts too. Think about your friends, family and workmates. How can you make their lives a little bit better? There will be one small thing that you can do for someone else that will improve their whole day. Perhaps if you know a colleague is hard pressed on a particular job you could leave a little treat on their desk first thing in the morning: a bunch of flowers or a small bar of chocolate could transform their day. Or perhaps you could help them tidy their desk. You might also like to make the tea or coffee more frequently than fairness dictates.

At home, you could do something that you know your partner hates doing. Or perhaps cook them their favourite food. You could babysit for a friend or neighbour. If you've finished a good book, why not leave it on a park bench or bus seat? Or donate it to a library. Why not do some 'de-cluttering' and get rid of your unwanted (or unneeded) possessions through a charity shop. You could also try 'freecycling' (freecycle.org and freegle.org are international movements that help you get rid of your old stuff by giving it away to people who need it and are willing to collect it).

We often hold back from helping others out of shyness or from fear of appearing foolish or even weak. If this is the case, focus on those fleeting sensations. Embrace them. Hold them for a moment before carrying on regardless. When it comes to kindness, be reckless.

CHAPTER ELEVEN

Week Eight: Life Lives Through You

'I received the letter in the post the other day. As soon as I saw the envelope I knew who it was from and decided to find a quiet space to have some time alone to absorb the words inside.'

Lotty had recently attended a mindfulness course, so she knew how to mentally prepare herself for the news inside that letter. Still, she needed a few moments to gather her thoughts and be ready for what it contained. She knew it might not make easy reading.

'I went to the downstairs loo – the only safe haven in my house where the boys don't think to look for me. Some women have a boudoir – I have a loo.

'I sat in my loo and slowly read the familiar handwriting on the pages. I reflected on the heartfelt, important and sage advice being conveyed and how essential it was for me take it all on board. You see, this letter was from me. No, I don't have multiple personalities and I haven't lost the plot. I had written the letter as the final exercise of a course that I attended on mindfulness – a course that has quite literally changed my life for the better. The letter was to consolidate all we had learned during our eight weeks. We were to write some words to remind ourselves of why it is important to be mindful and why it is necessary to make time for it.

'I had sealed the letter in an envelope and handed it to my teacher and she promised to post it back to me a month from then. This is what I wrote …

Dear Lotty
Life is too short and too precious to worry about the small things. Feel and be present in each moment so as not to waste it. If you are in pain, or it's a situation you don't want to be in, or it makes you anxious/stressed/unhappy, then either look at what you can do to change it, or change your reaction to it.

You are a good person in your heart who has great compassion and empathy for others and is capable of showing great tenderness. It is time to give some of that compassion and tenderness to yourself.

Liberate yourself from suffering and guilt – they serve you no purpose at all.

Take time to meditate every day, whether it is for five minutes or forty. It is important to your health and wellbeing and deserves a high priority in your life.

Think before you react in a difficult situation. Pause, breathe and make a better choice.

You deserve health, happiness, love, joy and everything

you ever dreamed of. You are surrounded by wealth and joy if you really look and appreciate it.

With loving kindness.

Lotty'

Lotty's letter to herself beautifully conveys the universal benefits of mindfulness. At the end of this chapter we'll invite you to write a similar letter to yourself, seal it in an envelope and ask a friend to post it back to you in a month's time. This will help you remember your reasons for continuing with your mindfulness practice.

Although this is the last week of the eight-week Mindfulness for Health programme, it is really the beginning of the rest of your life. In both respects, Week Eight is a milestone. In this chapter we'll review all that you've learned over the previous weeks and help you to find ways of maintaining your practice so that you can, if you choose, continue your journey of ever-deepening mindfulness.

As you've progressed through the course, you have learned three core mindfulness skills:

- **Focused awareness** – learning to pay attention to one thing at a time to cultivate a sense of calm stability.

- **Open monitoring** – learning to rest your mind in a broad and open field of awareness and to observe how your moment-to-moment experience of life constantly changes. This helps you to live a more harmonious life because you are perceiving it more accurately.

- **Loving kindness and compassion** – cultivating self-acceptance and care towards yourself and others. This reveals the similarities and connections between us all, dissolving stress and reactivity so that life becomes warm and wholesome once again.

However, in working through the programme, you may have lost sight of its overall structure, and how it was woven together, so here is a brief reminder:

During the first weeks of the programme you learned to focus your awareness on the breath and the body. You learned to give up your weight to gravity, rather than creating more tension by straining against it. As your practice deepened, the two types of suffering were gently teased apart and revealed: Primary and Secondary Suffering. Although Primary Suffering might be inevitable in the short term, Secondary Suffering is not. Most of the pain and distress that you actually *feel* is Secondary Suffering, and as this realisation became apparent, your suffering would have begun to lessen. The early weeks also revealed the mind's Doing mode. This is the logical, rational, problem-solving approach to the world. Although the Doing mode is one of humanity's greatest assets, it can create difficulties when it volunteers for a task that it simply cannot do, such as trying logically to 'solve' an emotion or troubling state of mind, or 'getting rid of' chronic pain or illness. This is one of the major driving forces behind Secondary Suffering and also the creation of anxiety, stress, depression and exhaustion. Switching to the mind's Being mode tends to dissolve these problems. Over the weeks you came to know that the Being mode is the state of pure awareness that lies behind all the clouds of thought and emotion. It allows you to see your thoughts as they appear in your mind, in all of their mercurial beauty. When you become aware of your 'negative' thoughts and emotions, they often melt away of their own accord along with any anxiety, stress, depression and suffering that you may be feeling. So you learned to look 'at' thoughts, rather than 'from' them. Through this you learned that thoughts are not facts – even some of those that claim to be.

You then moved on to extending the natural flow of the breath into the larger movements of the body through Mindful Movement exercises. These bring mindfulness into all the movements of daily life, both large and small. Next, you went on a journey to discover your own 'mindfulness rhythm' through pacing, to avoid slipping back into a boom-and-bust cycle, as well as helping to prevent over-stressing your body and mind.

As the weeks passed, you learned to counteract tendencies to be overly harsh or critical of yourself by cultivating a sense of acceptance and compassion towards yourself. And you learned to turn towards discomfort with kindness and tenderness. This helped you to accept, deep within your soul, the things that you cannot change (Primary Suffering) and to change those that you can (Secondary Suffering).

This, in turn, opened a door to the appreciation of pleasure once again. Reconnecting with the pleasant aspects of daily life was one of the most important skills you learned.

You then discovered how to broaden your awareness – like pulling back with a wide-angle lens on a camera – to create 'a bigger container' for your experiences. This gave you the capability to hold both pleasure and pain in the mind simultaneously, allowing you to see the fluid and changing nature of experience. And through this enhanced perspective, you learned to let go of the automatic tendency to push away pain and to cling on to pleasure and to live with more of a sense of 'flow'. This put an end to any struggle with the reality of life, so creating a sense of balance and stability.

But even this sense of warmth and compassion towards yourself was not *quite* enough. Although it transformed your suffering and stress, it was not quite sufficient for complete wellbeing. For this, you needed to widen your circle of compassion a little further to encompass other people. So you learned to expand the focus of your awareness from yourself to others. This helped to transform your perspective from one of separation and isolation to one of connection.

All of these steps allowed you to enact one of the central tenets of mindfulness: you cannot stop the world from changing, but you can influence your direction of travel by how you act. The direction you travel through life is your choice, even if the road is often winding and sometimes tortuous. So learning to *respond* to your own experiences – rather than *reacting* to them – with warmth and compassion, can lead to a richer and more fulfilling life. Reacting harshly simply leads to further difficulty and pain. It will take a lot of training for this attitude to fully permeate your life, but every second of mindfulness will help.

And this is where Week Eight begins: it is the start of the rest of your life. Through this you begin dissolving your remaining suffering and stress.

Practices for Week Eight

- Ten minutes of the Body Scan meditation (see page 63; track 1 on the CD), to be carried out on six days out of the next seven.
- Ten minutes of the Breathing Anchor meditation (see page 92; track 2 on the CD), to be carried out on six days out of the

next seven. You may also like to revisit some of the other meditations that seem especially relevant to you this week.

- Continue pacing with the Three-minute Breathing Space (see pages 215.
- Write a letter to yourself (see page 219).

Once this week's formal meditations are over, you will need a reason to continue with your practice. After all, you are investing that most precious commodity in the fast-paced world we live in: time. It is sensible to think about your reason now, otherwise your practice will tend to get squeezed out by other, seemingly higher, priorities. So spend a few moments considering why you wish to continue with your practice. You might like to close your eyes …

… and think …

Imagine dropping a stone down a deep well and listening for the echoes. Those echoes might contain the deepest reasons for you to continue. They might include:

- keeping pain under control
- living a fulfilling life while still in pain
- reducing stress and overall unhappiness
- doing it for your family
- being able to remain calm and energised

- remaining freer from anger, bitterness and cynicism
- being able to live each day with appreciation and openness.

Here we invite you to examine your deepest reasons and desires for maintaining your practice. Some find that one or more of the reasons we've just outlined are sufficient. Others need to delve a little deeper.

Whatever reasons you unearth for continuing with your practice, you will need to decide on the meditations that are sustainable for *you* in the long term. Remember that your choices are not set in stone. They can change from day to day and from year to year. Sometimes you might feel the need to simply focus on the breath and the body with the Body Scan (see page 63) or Breathing Anchor (see page 92). Other times you might feel a sense of isolation and want to reconnect with life through the Connection meditation (see page 205). If your pain or stress should flare up again, then the Compassionate Acceptance meditation might be especially helpful (see page 134). Feel free to weave these practices together in whatever manner you find most helpful.

So how long should you meditate for?

Allow the practice itself to tell you. Most days you should consider meditating for ten to twenty minutes. Some days you might like to practise for longer (you will find longer meditations at www.breathworks.org.uk and www.franticworld.com). When considering how long you should meditate for, bear in mind that one of the words that translate into English as 'meditation' from the original Pali language also means 'cultivation'. Meditation, like a crop of fine fruit, cannot be rushed. It is a process that unfolds over many months and years. It needs tending to most days. If you still need to know how long to meditate for, why not go into the orchard of your mind and see for yourself?

Yoga teachers say that the most difficult move of all is getting on to the mat. Remember this when you meet resistance to your practice. Simply begin. Agree with yourself that you will meditate for just one minute . . . Often as not, you will find yourself meditating for longer.

Whichever meditations you choose, be creative and flexible. Each time you practise, see if you can approach them with a sense of freshness and wonder. There is a delightful phrase for this fresh and innocent awareness: 'beginner's mind'. This attitude will help you to maintain your humility and readiness to learn. It is summed up by the Zen teacher Shunryu Suzuki, who said: 'In the beginner's mind there are many possibilities, but in the expert's there are few.' [1]

Remember also that mindfulness is much more than the ten-minute meditations you have found in this book. It is the quality of awareness that you bring to your whole life. You might find it useful to develop your own mindfulness 'toolkit', drawing on everything you've learned – something you can keep in reserve to use if suffering should return or if life should begin slipping through your fingers. You'll find ideas for this in the box below.

Mindfulness Toolkit

It's always useful to have an emergency 'toolkit' on hand containing all you need to get your life back on track again when things begin to go awry. And it's important that this is pre-prepared so that everything is ready should the need arise.

Take some time to sit quietly and bring to mind the techniques and ideas from the programme that you have found most useful. Write them down. The idea is to create a list of ideas, phrases and techniques that will make you stop, pause and become a little more mindful. The list should also include a few short practices that will encourage you to re-engage with life – and mindfulness – once again.

Choose as many 'tools' as you like. You could take one from each week of the programme, plus a couple of extras; or perhaps a handful that you have found most useful. Include a range of ideas and practices that will cover most of the situations you are likely to find yourself in. And to pre-empt potential dithering, state near the top of the list: 'Stuck? Choose something at random!'

Once you have prepared your toolkit you might like to carry it around with you or, perhaps, pin it up somewhere that you'll see it regularly. Remember also to review your toolkit from time to time. You may discover that some new elements have come to the fore.

Here are some items that you might like to include:

- Take a Three-minute Breathing Space: don't forget to stop regularly in daily life and come back to focusing on the breathing body.
- Remember 'thoughts are not facts' and to look 'at' thoughts, not 'from' them. Don't take your thoughts and emotions so seriously – particularly negative ones.
- Take a break before you need it. Remember to pace yourself.

- Remember the difference between Primary and Secondary Suffering.
- Notice the pleasant. Ask yourself, 'How many pleasant things can I notice in this moment?'
- Is this the Doing mode talking? Is it volunteering for a task it cannot do?
- Smile, even if it's forced. Breathe. Is there tension in the shoulders, neck, arms, hands . . . ?
- Begin the day with mindfulness. When you open your eyes, take in the scene . . . the ceiling, the walls . . . What can you feel, hear, smell . . . ?
- Move slowly. Be aware of your movement and of the breath.
- Befriend your feelings. Bring kind-hearted awareness to even your most difficult emotions.
- When you feel tired, frustrated, stressed, anxious, in pain – or have any difficult feeling or sensation – stop and take a Breathing Space.
- Mindful movement: do some mindful movements, even if it is only a minute of rolling your shoulders.
- Remember that happiness and sadness are twins; they co-exist in us all and both eventually melt away.
- Mindful action: whatever you are doing in this moment, do it mindfully, with full awareness.
- Be a yacht, not a dinghy. Sail calmly through the waves of life, rather than being tossed about by the ocean swell.

- Remember the three Cs – Care, Compassion and Commitment to life as it is, rather than as you want it to be.
- Relax tension: is there any tension in the jaw, shoulders, neck, hands or anywhere else? Breathe into it to soften tension.
- Don't become trapped in the past or future. All thoughts are transient. Let them pass.
- *Act*, rather than *react*, towards powerful thoughts and emotions. When you sense them building, broaden your awareness.
- Is a sense of resistance building? To what? Want to be elsewhere, anywhere but here right now? Soften, be kind. If you feel numb, zoom in. If you feel overwhelmed, zoom out.
- Remember to *accept* things that you can't change immediately; or *change* them if you can. Just take one step. Be kind to your feelings of 'non-acceptance'. Embrace them. Promise to take another look at the situation tomorrow, next week, month or next year.
- Remember, your breath is always with you.
- Think of others. Commit a random act of kindness.
- Stop, breathe and remember how connected we all are.
- Have a cup of tea, a biscuit, and sit down for five minutes.

Whichever practices you eventually settle upon, try to make sure that you maintain your mindfulness rhythm in daily life and continue to pace yourself if you've found this useful. You will probably find that you will gradually be able to extend your baselines, but be careful of slipping into a boom-and-bust cycle. When it comes to baselines, be prudent.

As your mindfulness practice deepens over the coming months and years, you will find that the Three-minute Breathing Space becomes one of your closest friends. When the world is falling apart, when suffering and stress seem insurmountable, when depression and exhaustion loom ever larger, it will always pay to punctuate your day with a few Breathing Spaces. It is also a gentle way of keeping in touch with your baselines. If you take only one thing from this course, let it be the Breathing Space.

And what of the Habit Releasers? Habitual ways of thinking and behaving tend to lock suffering in place, so gently loosening their grip should become a regular part of your life. By now you will have learned that this can be as simple as stopping for a few moments and releasing your weight to gravity, making a cup of tea for a friend (and letting the kettle boil until it clicks off), taking a different route to work or watching a sunset from a park bench. Simply altering your routine ways of doing things will help to reduce the stress and tension that exacerbate suffering. It will allow you to move away from the autopilot and the habitual and compulsive 'Doing' mode, and towards living with choice and the 'Being' mode. Habit Releasers are a wonderfully simple way of incorporating mindful awareness into daily life. So if you take a second thing from this course, let it be habit releasing.

FINDING TRUE WELLBEING

When you are suffering with chronic pain, illness or stress, life can become intolerable. It can seem as if the world is conspiring against you – almost as if it has been designed from the ground up to make your life as difficult as possible. In your darkest hours, feelings of hopelessness and despair can arise. But it is precisely in these hours that the greatest lessons can be learned. For if you can learn to step aside from the fray for a few moments, long enough to take a single breath, then you can catch a glimpse of a better way of living. If you can smile inwardly to yourself, show yourself a little kindness, then you start to create a tiny current within you that flows towards greater awareness and compassion. In this way, every moment of awareness is like a drop of morning dew that adds to a stream. Eventually this stream grows into a tiny brook ... a river. And after a while, the current becomes so naturally strong that warmth and compassion towards yourself – and others – simply becomes a natural state of affairs. This warmth dissolves suffering and stress, leaving behind a true sense of wellbeing.

WRITING YOURSELF A LETTER

Now, finally, you can write yourself a letter. It can be like Lotty's or completely different. There is no template – no 'right' or 'wrong' way. Simply write the letter that you'd love to receive, reminding yourself of all the things you've gained from this course, and maybe mentioning all your qualities and ideals. We give you a completely blank canvas. Nobody else need see what you've written.

Once you've written your letter, seal it in an envelope, put a stamp on it and give it to a friend to post back to you in a month's time.

Whatever happens, whatever you write, remember these words from the Nobel laureate Derek Walcott:

Love After Love

The time will come
when, with elation
you will greet yourself arriving
at your own door, in your own mirror
and each will smile at the other's welcome,

and say, sit here. Eat.
You will love again the stranger who was your self.
Give wine. Give bread. Give back your heart
to itself, to the stranger who has loved you

all your life, whom you ignored
for another, who knows you by heart.
Take down the love letters from the bookshelf,

the photographs, the desperate notes,
peel your own image from the mirror.
Sit. Feast on your life.

NOTES

CHAPTER ONE

1. Brown, Christopher A., Jones, Anthony K. P., (2013) 'Psychobiological Correlates of Improved Mental Health in Patients With Musculoskeletal Pain After a Mindfulness-based Pain Management Program', *Clinical Journal of Pain*, 29(3), pp. 233–44.
2. Baer, R. A., Smith, G. T., Hopkins, J., Kreitemeyer, J. & Toney, L. (2006), 'Using self-report assessment methods to explore facets of mindfulness', *Assessment,* 13, pp. 27–45.
3. Brown, Christopher A., Jones, Anthony K. P., (2013) 'Psychobiological Correlates of Improved Mental Health in Patients With Musculoskeletal Pain After a Mindfulness-based Pain Management Program', *Clinical Journal of Pain*, 29(3), pp. 233–44.
4. Zeidan, F., Martucci, K. T., Kraft, R. A., Gordon, N. S., McHaffie, J. G. & Coghill, R. C. 2011, 'Brain Mechanisms Supporting the Modulation of Pain by Mindfulness Meditation', *Journal of Neuroscience*, 31(14), p. 5540. See also the accompanying comments regarding morphine effectiveness by Fadel Zeidan of the Wake Forest University School of Medicine at http://ow.ly/i8rZs.
5. Kabat-Zinn, J., Lipworth, L., Burncy, R. & Sellers, W. (1986), 'Four-year follow-up of a meditation-based program for the self- regulation of chronic pain: Treatment outcomes and compliance', *Clinical Journal of Pain*, 2, p. 159; Morone, N. E., Greco, C. M. & Weiner, D. K. (2008), 'Mindfulness meditation for the treatment of chronic

low back pain in older adults: A randomized controlled pilot study', *Pain*, 134(3), pp. 310–19; Grant, J. A. & Rainville, P. (2009), 'Pain sensitivity and analgesic effects of mindful states in zen meditators: A cross-sectional study', *Psychosomatic Medicine*, 71(1), pp. 106–14.

6. Brown, Christopher A., Jones, Anthony K. P. 2013, MD, 'Psychobiological Correlates of Improved Mental Health in Patients With Musculoskeletal Pain After a Mindfulness-based Pain Management Program', *Clinical Journal of Pain*, 29(3), pp. 233–44.
7. Zeidan, F., Martucci, K. T., Kraft, R. A., Gordon, N. S., McHaffie, J. G. & Coghill, R. C. 2011, 'Brain Mechanisms Supporting the Modulation of Pain by Mindfulness Meditation', *Journal of Neuroscience*, 31(14), p. 5540. See also the accompanying comments regarding morphine effectiveness by Fadel Zeidan of the Wake Forest University School of Medicine at http://ow.ly/i8rZs.
8. Grossman, P., Tiefenthaler-Gilmer, U., Raysz, A. & Kesper, U. (2007), 'Mindfulness training as an intervention for fibromyalgia: evidence of postintervention and 3-year follow-up benefits in well-being', *Psychotherapy and Psychosomatics*, 76, pp. 226–233; Sephton, S. E., Salmon, P., Weissbecker, I., Ulmer, C., Floyd, A., Hoover, K., et al. (2007), 'Mindfulness meditation alleviates depressive symptoms in women with fibromyalgia: results of a randomized clinical trial', *Arthritis & Rheumatism*, 57, pp. 77–85; Schmidt, S., Grossman, P., Schwarzer, B., Jena, S., Naumann, J., and Walach, H. (2011), 'Treating fibromyalgia with mindfulness-based stress reduction: results from a 3-armed randomized controlled trial', *Pain* 152, pp. 361–9.
9. Morone, N. E., Lynch, C. S., Greco, C. M., Tindle, H. A. & Weiner, D. K. (2008b), '"I felt like a new person" – the effects of mindfulness meditation on older adults with chronic pain: qualitative narrative analysis of diary entries', *Journal of Pain*, 9, pp. 841–8.
10. Gaylord, S. A., Palsson, O. S., Garland, E. L., Faurot, K. R., Coble, R. S., Mann, J. D., et al. (2011), 'Mindfulness training reduces the severity of irritable bowel syndrome in women: results of a randomized controlled trial', *American Journal of Gastroenterology*, 106, pp. 1678–88.
11. Grossman, P., Kappos, L., Gensicke, H., D'souza, M., Mohr, D. C., Penner, I. K., et al. (2010), 'MS quality of life, depression, and fatigue improve after mindfulness training: a randomized trial', *Neurology*, 75, pp. 1141–9.

12. Speca, M., Carlson, L., Goodey, E. & Angen, M. (2000), 'A randomized, wait-list controlled clinical trial: the effect of a mindfulness meditation-based stress reduction program on mood and symptoms of stress in cancer outpatients', *Psychosomatic Medicine*, 62, pp. 613–22.
13. Jha, A., et al. (2007), 'Mindfulness training modifies subsystems of attention', *Cognitive Affective and Behavioral Neuroscience*, 7, pp. 109–19; Tang, Y. Y., Ma, Y., Wang, J., Fan, Y., Feng, S., Lu, Q., et al. (2007), 'Short-term meditation training improves attention and self-regulation', *Proceedings of the National Academy of Sciences (US)*, 104(43), pp. 17152–6. McCracken, L. M. & Yang, S.-Y. (2008), 'A contextual cognitive-behavioral analysis of rehabilitation workers' health and well-being: Influences of acceptance, mindfulness and values-based action', *Rehabilitation Psychology*, 53, pp.479–85; Ortner, C. N. M., Kilner, S. J. & Zelazo, P. D. (2007), 'Mindfulness meditation and reduced emotional interference on a cognitive task', *Motivation and Emotion*, 31, pp. 271–83; Brefczynski-Lewis, J. A., Lutz, A., Schaefer, H. S., Levinson, D. B. & Davidson, R. J. (2007), 'Neural correlates of attentional expertise in long-term meditation practitioners', *Proceedings of the National Academy of Sciences (US)*, 104(27), pp. 11483–8.
14. Brown, Kirk Warren, Ryan, Richard, M. (2003), 'The benefits of being present: Mindfulness and its role in psychological well-being', *Journal of Personality and Social Psychology*, 84(4), pp. 822–48; Lykins, Emily L. B. & Baer, Ruth A. (2009), 'Psychological Functioning in a Sample of Long-Term Practitioners of Mindfulness Meditation', *Journal of Cognitive Psychotherapy*, 23(3), pp. 226–41.
15. Ivanowski, B. & Malhi, G. S. (2007), 'The psychological and neurophysiological concomitants of mindfulness forms of meditation', *Acta Neuropsychiatrica,* 19, pp. 76–91; Shapiro, S. L., Oman, D., Thoresen, C. E., Plante, T. G. & Flinders, T. (2008), 'Cultivating mindfulness: effects on well-being', *Journal of Clinical Psychology*, 64(7), pp. 840–62; Shapiro, S. L., Schwartz, G. E. & Bonner, G. (1998), 'Effects of mindfulness-based stress reduction on medical and premedical students', *Journal of Behavioral Medicine,* 21, pp. 581–99.
16. See NICE Guidelines for Management of Depression (2004, 2009). Ma, J. & Teasdale, J. D. (2004), 'Mindfulness-based cognitive therapy for depression: Replication and exploration of differential relapse prevention effects', *Journal of Consulting and Clinical Psychology,* 72, pp. 31–40; Segal, Z. V., Williams, J. M. G. & Teasdale, J. D.,

Mindfulness-based Cognitive Therapy for Depression: a new approach to preventing relapse (Guilford Press, 2002); Kenny, M. A. & Williams, J. M. G. (2007), 'Treatment-resistant depressed patients show a good response to Mindfulness-Based Cognitive Therapy', *Behaviour Research & Therapy*, 45, pp. 617–25; Eisendraeth, S. J., Delucchi, K., Bitner, R., Fenimore, P., Smit, M. & McLane, M. (2008), 'Mindfulness-Based Cognitive Therapy for Treatment-Resistant Depression: A Pilot Study', *Psychotherapy and Psychosomatics*, 77, pp. 319–20; Kingston, T., et al. (2007), 'Mindfulness-based cognitive therapy for residual depressive symptoms', *Psychology and Psychotherapy*, 80, pp. 193–203.

17. Bowen, S., et al. (2006), 'Mindfulness Meditation and Substance Use in an Incarcerated Population', *Psychology of Addictive Behaviors*, 20, pp. 343–7.
18. Hölzel, B. K., Ott, U., Gard, T., Hempel, H., Weygandt, M., Morgen, K. & Vaitl, D. (2008), 'Investigation of mindfulness meditation practitioners with voxel-based morphometry', *Social Cognitive and Affective Neuroscience*, 3, pp 55–61; Lazar, S., Kerr, C., Wasserman, R., Gray, J., Greve, D., Treadway, M., McGarvey, M., Quinn, B., Dusek, J., Benson, H., Rauch, S., Moore, C. & Fischl, B. (2005), 'Meditation experience is associated with increased cortical thickness', *NeuroReport*, 16, pp. 1893–7; Luders, Eileen, Toga, Arthur W., Lepore, Natasha & Gaser, Christian (2009), 'The underlying anatomical correlates of long-term meditation: Larger hippocampal and frontal volumes of gray matter', *Neuroimage*, 45, pp. 672–8.
19. Tang, Y., Ma, Y., Wang, J., Fan, Y., Feg, S., Lu, Q., Yu, Q., Sui, D., Rothbart, M., Fan, M. & Posner, M. (2007), 'Short-term meditation training improves attention and self-regulation', *Proceedings of the National Academy of Sciences*, 104, pp. 17152–6.
20. Davidson, R. J. (2004), 'Well-being and affective style: Neural substrates and biobehavioural correlates', *Philosophical Transactions of the Royal Society*, 359, pp. 1395–1411.
21. Lazar, S., Kerr, C., Wasserman, R., Gray, J., Greve, D., Treadway, M., McGarvey, M., Quinn, B., Dusek, J., Benson, J., Rauch, S., Moore, C. & Fischl, B. (2005), 'Meditation experience is associated with increased cortical thickness', *NeuroReport*, 16, pp 1893–7.
22. Davidson, R. J., Kabat-Zinn, J. Schumacher, J., Rosenkranz, M., Muller, D., Santorelli, S.F., Urbanowski, F., Harrington, A., Bonus, K. & Sheridan, J. F. (2003) 'Alterations in brain and immune function produced by mindfulness meditation', *Psychosomatic Medicine*, 65,

pp. 564–70; Tang, Y., Ma, Y., Wang, J., Fan, Y., Feg, S., Lu, Q., Yu, Q., Sui, D., Rothbart, M., Fan, M. & Posner, M. (2007), 'Short-term meditation training improves attention and self-regulation', *Proceedings of the National Academy of Sciences*, 104, pp. 17152–6.

23. Epel, Elissa, Daubenmier, Jennifer, Tedlie Moskowitz, Judith, Folkman, Susan & Blackburn, Elizabeth (2009), 'Can Meditation Slow Rate of Cellular Aging? Cognitive Stress, Mindfulness, and Telomeres', *Annals of the New York Academy of Sciences*, 1172; *Longevity, Regeneration, and Optimal Health Integrating Eastern and Western Perspectives*, pp. 34–53.
24. Walsh, R. & Shapiro, S. L. (2006), 'The meeting of meditative disciplines and Western psychology: A mutually enriching dialogue', *American Psychologist*, 61, pp. 227–39.
25. Ibid.
26. Kabat-Zinn, J., Lipworth, L., Burncy, R. & Sellers, W. (1986), 'Four-year follow-up of a meditation-based program for the self- regulation of chronic pain: Treatment outcomes and compliance', *Clinical Journal of Pain*, 2, p. 159; Brown, Christopher A., Jones, Anthony K. P. (2013), 'Psychobiological Correlates of Improved Mental Health in Patients With Musculoskeletal Pain After a Mindfulness-based Pain Management Program', *Clinical Journal of Pain*, 29(3), pp. 233–44; Lutz, Antoine, McFarlin, Daniel R., Perlman, David M., Salomons, Tim V. & Davidson, Richard J. (2013), 'Altered anterior insula activation during anticipation and experience of painful stimuli in expert meditators', *Journal NeuroImage*, 64, pp. 538–46.
27. Baliki, Marwan N., Bogdan, Petre, Torbey, Souraya, Herrmann, Kristina M., Huang, Leijan, Schnitzer, Thomas J., Fields, Howard L. &, Vania Apkarian, A. (2012), 'Corticostriatal functional connectivity predicts transition to chronic back pain', *Nature* Neuroscience, 15, pp. 1117–19.
28. Adapted from *Mindfulness: A practical guide to finding peace in a frantic world*, by Mark Williams and Danny Penman.

CHAPTER TWO

1. Wall, Patrick D. & Ronald Melzack, *The Challenge of Pain* (Penguin Books, 1982), p. 98; Melzack, R. Wall, p. D. (1965), 'Pain Mechanisms: a new theory, *Science*, 150(3699), pp. 371–9.
2. Cole, Frances, Macdonald, Helen, Carus, Catherine & Howden-Leach,

Hazel, *Overcoming Chronic Pain* (Constable & Robinson, 2005), p. 37; Bond, M., Simpson, K., Pain: Its Nature and Treatment (Elsevier, 2006), p. 16, offers an alternative definition from the International Association for the Study of Pain as acute pain (lasting less than one month), sub-acute pain (lasting one to six months) and chronic pain (lasting six months or more).
3. 'Health Survey for England 2011', Health, social care and lifestyles, Chapter 9 Chronic Pain, The Health and Social Care Information Centre (NHS) 20 December 2012, www.ic.nhs.uk/catalogue/PUB09300.
4. Gaskin, Darrell J. & Richard, Patrick (2012), 'The Economic Costs of Pain in the United States', *Journal of Pain*, 13(8), p. 715.
5. 'Health Survey for England 2011', Health, social care and lifestyles, Chapter 9 Chronic Pain, The Health and Social Care Information Centre (NHS) 20 December 2012, www.ic.nhs.uk/catalogue/PUB09300.
6. NOP Pain Survey (2005), 23–25 September, on behalf of the British Pain Society.
7. Ploghaus, Alexander, Narain, Charvy, Beckmann, Christian F., Clare, Stuart, Bantick, Susanna, Wise, Richard, Matthews, Paul M., Nicholas, J., Rawlins, P. & Tracey, Irene (2001), 'Exacerbation of Pain by Anxiety Is Associated with Activity in a Hippocampal Network', *Journal of Neuroscience*, 21(24), pp. 9896–903.
8. Zeidan, Fadel, Martucci, Katherine T., Kraft, Robert A., Gordon, Nakia S., McHaffie, John G. & Coghill, Robert C. (2011), 'Brain Mechanisms Supporting the Modulation of Pain by Mindfulness Meditation', *Journal of Neuroscience*, 31(14), pp. 5540–48. See also the accompanying comments regarding morphine effectiveness by Fadel Zeidan of the Wake Forest University School of Medicine at http://ow.ly/i8rZs.

CHAPTER FOUR

1. Donna Farhi, *The Breathing Book*, (Harry Holt and Company, 1996).
2. Roberts, Monty, *The Man Who Listens to Horses* (Arrow Books, 1997).

CHAPTER FIVE

1. Zindel V. Segal, J., Mark G. Williams, John Teasdale, *Mindfulness-Based Cognitive Therapy for Depression: A New Approach to*

Preventing Relapse, The Guildford Press (New York), 2002 (see p. 73).

2. Ibid.
3. Zeidan, F., Grant, J. A., Brown, C. A., McHaffie, J. G., Coghill, R. C. (2012), 'Mindfulness meditation-related pain relief: Evidence for unique brain mechanisms in the regulation of pain', *Neuroscience Letters* 520, pp. 165–173. See also: Brown, C. A., Jones, A. K. P., 'Meditation experience predicts less negative appraisal of pain: Electrophysiological evidence for the involvement of anticipatory neural responses', *PAIN* (2010), doi:10.1016/j.pain.2010.04.017. See also its accompanying commentary by Buhle, J. (2010), 'Does meditation training lead to enduring changes in the anticipation and experience of pain?' *PAIN* 150, pp. 382–383.

CHAPTER SIX

1. Dickstein, Ruth, Deutsch, Judith E. (2007), 'Motor Imagery in Physical Therapist Practice', *Physical Therapy*, 87(7), American Physical Therapy Association, July 2007, pp. 942–53.

CHAPTER SEVEN

1. As an example: Desbordes, Gaële, Negl, Lobsang T., Pace, Thaddeus W. W., Wallace, B. Alan, Raison, Charles L., & Schwartz, Eric L (2012), 'Effects of mindful-attention and compassion meditation training on amygdala response to emotional stimuli in an ordinary, non-meditative state', *Frontiers in Human Neuroscience Journal*, 6:29, doi:10.3389/fnhum.2012.00292

CHAPTER EIGHT

1. Hanson, R., *Buddah's Brain: The Practical Neuroscience of Happiness, Love and Wisdom*, (New Harbinger Publications, 2009).
2. Gilbert, Paul, *The Compassionate Mind* (Constable, 2010 edition); first published 2009; paperback edition published 2010, p. 34.
3. From 'This' by Maitreyabandhu, *The Crumb Road* (Bloodaxe Books, 2013).

CHAPTER NINE

1. From the poem 'Kindness' by Naomi Shihab Nye.
2. Originally coined by Dacher Keltner, PhD and now used increasingly by other leading social scientists.
3. For a good overview see Chapter Two of *The Compassionate Mind* by Paul Gilbert (Constable & Robinson, 2009).
4. Adapted from Chapter Two *The Compassionate Mind* by Paul Gilbert (Constable & Robinson, 2009).
5. Costa, Joana & Pinto-Gouveia, José (2011), 'Acceptance of Pain, Self-Compassion and Psychopathology: Using the Chronic Pain Acceptance Questionnaire to Identify Patients' Subgroups', *Clinical Psychology and Psychotherapy*, 18, pp. 292–302.
6. Carson, J. W., Keefe, F. J., Lynch, T. R., et al. (2005), 'Loving- kindness meditation for chronic low back pain: results from a pilot trial', *Journal of Holistic Nursing*, 23, pp. 287–304.
7. Thaddeus, W. W., et al. (2009), 'Effect of compassion meditation on neuroendocrine, innate immune and behavioral responses to psychosocial stress', *Psychoneuroendocrinology*, 34, pp. 87–98.
8. A good overview of the evidence is provided by Halifax, J. (2011), 'The Precious Necessity of Compassion', *Journal of Pain and Symptom Management*, 41(1), pp. 146–53.
9. Wren, Anava A., et al. (2012), 'Self-Compassion in Patients With Persistent Musculoskeletal Pain: Relationship of Self-Compassion to Adjustment to Persistent Pain', *Journal of Pain and Symptom Management*, 43(4), pp. 759–70.
10. 'The Compassionate Brain' audio series, 'Session 1: How the Mind Changes the Brain', www.SoundsTrue.com, 2012. An interview between Dr Rick Hanson and Dr Richard Davison.
11. In the Buddhist meditative tradition 'focused awareness' is known as *samatha* and 'open monitoring' is known as *vipassana*.

CHAPTER TEN

1. Quote taken from Calaprice, Alice (ed.) *Dear Professor Einstein: Albert Einstein's Letters to and from Children* (Princeton University Press, 2002).
2. Stout, C., Morrow, J., Brandt, E. N., Wolf, S. (1964), 'Study of an Italian-American community in PA; unusually low incidence of death from myocardial infarction', *JAMA*, pp. 188:845–49.

3. Egolf, B., Lasker, J., Wolf, S. & Potvin, L. (1992), 'The Roseto effect: a 50-year comparison of mortality rates, *American Journal of Public Health*, 82(8), pp. 1089–92.
4. Fredrickson, Barbara L., Coffey, Kimberly A., Pek, Jolynn, Cohn, Michael A., Finkel & Sandra M. (2008), 'Open Hearts Build Lives: Positive Emotions, Induced Through Loving-Kindness Meditation, Build Consequential Personal Resources', *Journal of Personality and Social Psychology,* 95(5), pp. 1045–62,
5. Adapted from Mindfulness-Based Cognitive Therapy (MBCT). See Segal, Zindel V., Williams, J. Mark G. & Teasdale, John, *Mindfulness-Based Cognitive Therapy for Depression: A New Approach to Preventing Relapse* (The Guildford Press, 2002), p. 241.

CHAPTER ELEVEN

1. Shunryu Suzuki, *Zen Mind, Beginners' Mind* (Weatherhill, 1973), epigraph.

RESOURCES

MEDITATION EQUIPMENT

Mindfulness and meditation practice are easier to maintain if you have aids that help you to be as comfortable as possible. The following items may help.

- For lying-down postures: a meditation or yoga mat for comfort; a yoga bolster, which can help to ease pressure on the spine if placed under the knees; and an eye-bag, which can help the eyes relax.
- If you kneel or sit on the floor to meditate try one of the following: a meditation cushion (sometimes called a zafu); a meditation stool (a small wooden stool to slide your knees under); or yoga blocks (2 blocks – 305mm x 205mm x 50mm is a good size). A rubber stability cushion (inflated to the correct height and placed on top of the yoga blocks) is also a good way to take the strain off the spine and sacrum. These are marketed as 'stability cushions', 'wobble cushions', 'balance cushions' or 'airdisks'.

- If you sit on a chair to meditate make sure you use a straight-backed chair such as a dining chair. You may find it helpful to place a meditation cushion/zafu beneath the feet, and a stability cushion can help relieve pressure under the sacrum and sitting bones.

Contact Breathworks at info@breathworks.co.uk for details of how to buy these items, or search the Internet for local suppliers if you live outside the UK. You can access vidoes showing different meditation postures and equipment at www.breathworks-mindfulness.org.uk or www.franticworld.com.

MINDFUL MOVEMENT

The mindful movements in this book are part of a larger programme developed by Breathworks. If you are interested in learning the full range of movements please contact info@breathworks.co.uk and enquire about the 'mindful movement' pack.

MINDFULNESS IN DAILY LIFE

It helps to invest in a timer to help you with your pacing/rhythm. Any digital countdown timer will do, but ideally find a product that has at least two rotating cycles so you can alternate activity and rest cycles, e.g. 15 minutes working and 5 minutes lying down on a continuous rotating cycle. Timex Ironman watches have this feature (called a countdown interval timer) and the Enzo clock is also very good http://www.salubrion.com/products/ensoclock/.

BREATHWORKS COURSES

There are a variety of ways to support your learning as you follow the course in this book. Through Breathworks you can do it in a group with others, or join an online group. Individual tuition and support is also available. You can also train to become a Breathworks mindfulness teacher and offer the programme to others. For a list of accredited Breathworks teachers and details about learning opportunities visit www.breathworks-mindfulness.org.uk

OTHER RELEVANT WEBSITES

www.franticworld.com The website to accompany the sister volume to this book: *Mindfulness: a practical guide to finding peace in a frantic world*. It also contains resources to complement this volume and a forum to discuss your experiences and to learn from others. There are links to further meditations and books that you might find useful, plus a section listing upcoming talks, events and retreats.

www.mindfulnessteachersuk.org.uk This website contains information about the UK Network for Mindfulness-based Teacher Training Organisations, who are committed to supporting good practice and integrity in the delivery of mindfulness-based courses in the UK. The network is supported by all the main training organisations in the UK who train teachers to deliver mindfulness-based courses.

www.umassmed.edu/cfm This is the website for the Center for Mindfulness at the University of Massachusetts Medical School. This organisation pioneered bringing mindfulness into healthcare and was founded by Dr Jon Kabat-Zinn. You can also find tapes/CDs of meditation practices recorded by Jon Kabat-Zinn at **www.stressreductiontapes.com.**

ONLINE MEDITATION INSTRUCTION AND RESOURCES

www.wildmind.org This site offers a comprehensive programme of online meditation instruction and support. It also stocks a wide range of CDs of led practices.

www.thebuddhistcentre.com The website for Triratna Buddhist Community – the organisation that Vidyamala practises within.

For more information on the dialogue between modern science and Buddhism, please visit the Mind & Life Institute at **www.investigatingthemind.org.**

RETREATS

A residential retreat is an ideal way to consolidate your learning and practice in supportive and beautiful conditions. There are many retreat centres offering a range of events in many countries. You will find more information on the Internet. Here are a couple of examples:
www.goingonretreat.com
www.gaiahouse.co.uk

AUSTRALIAN AND NEW ZEALAND RESOURCES

Breathworks
www.breathworks-mindfulness.net This website contains details of Breathworks courses in Sydney.

Interest groups

MBSR-MBCT ANZ@yahoogroups.com is an online group established by a Sydney-based MBCT teacher, Chrissie Burke, who updates members regularly with news of relevant conferences, research articles and mindfulness events. Members can ask questions, network and collaborate. To join the list of members email Chrissie (chrissie.burke@gmail.com).

Meditation centres

www.sydneybuddhistcentre.org.au
www.melbournebuddhistcentre.org.au
www.dharma.org.au

Other online resources of interest

www.openground.com.au For information on mindfulness courses and training around Australia.

www.mindfulexperience.org The home of The Mindfulness Research Guide, a comprehensive resource that:

1. Provides information to researchers and practitioners on the scientific study of mindfulness, including research publications, measurement tools and mindfulness research centres.
2. Hosts the Mindfulness Research monthly bulletin for the purpose of keeping researchers and practitioners informed of current advances in research.

FURTHER READING

Vidyamala and Danny have both written other books that are relevant to the material in this book:

Burch, V., *Living Well with Pain & Illness – Using mindfulness to free yourself from suffering* (Piatkus, 2008). This is Vidyamala's first book and goes deeply into the themes of using mindfulness to live well with pain and illness. This is recommended further reading.

Williams, M., & Penman D., *Mindfulness: A practical guide to finding peace in a frantic world* (Piatkus, 2011). Published by Rodale in the US and Canada as *Mindfulness: An eight-week plan for finding peace in a frantic world.* This is the sister volume to *Mindfulness for Health,* written by Danny and Professor Mark Williams. It includes an eight-week programme to help you break the cycle of unhappiness, stress, anxiety and mental exhaustion that may be inhibiting your life. We also recommend this as further reading.

The selection below is meant as an introduction and as an invitation to explore. Many of these teachers and authors have written more books than are listed here and have meditation tapes/CDs you can buy.

MEDITATION, HEALTH AND PSYCHOLOGY

Bennett-Goleman, T., *Emotional Alchemy: How the Mind Can Heal the Heart* (Harmony Books, 2001).

Bertherat T. & Bernstein C., *The Body Has its Reasons* (Healing Arts Press, 1989).

Brazier, C., *A Buddhist psychology: Liberate your mind, embrace life* (Robinson Publishing, 2003).

Crane, R., *Mindfulness-based Cognitive Therapy* (Routledge, 2008).

Dahl, J., & Lundgren T., *Living Beyond Your Pain* (New Harbinger Publications, 2006).

Epstein, M., *Going on Being: Buddhism and the Way of Change, a Positive Psychology for the West* (Broadway Books, 2001).

Epstein, M., *Going to Pieces without Falling Apart: A Buddhist Perspective on Wholeness* (*Thorsons*, 1999).

Epstein, M., *Thoughts without a Thinker: psychotherapy from a Buddhist perspective* (Basic Books, 2005).

Farhi, D., *The Breathing Book* (Henry Holt & Company, 1996).

Germer, C., *The Mindful Path to Self-Compassion: Freeing Yourself from Destructive Thoughts and Emotions* (Guilford Press, 2009).

Gilbert, P., *The Compassionate Mind: A New Approach to Life's Challenges* (Constable & Robinson Limited, 2010).

Gilbert, P. & Chodon, *Mindful Compassion* (Robinson, 2013).

Goleman, D., *Destructive Emotions: How Can We Overcome Them? A Scientific Dialogue with the Dalai Lama* (Bantam Books, 2004).

Goleman, D., *Emotional Intelligence* (Bantam Books, 1995).

Goleman, D., *Working with Emotional Intelligence* (Bantam Books, 1998).

Kabat-Zinn, J., *Coming to Our Senses (*Piatkus, 2005).

Kabat-Zinn, J., *Full Catastrophe Living* (Piatkus, 2001).

Klein, A., *Chronic Pain: The Complete Guide to Relief* (Carroll & Graf Publishing, 2001).

Kubler-Ross, E., *On Death and Dying* (Simon and Schuster, 1997).

Levine, S., *Healing into Life and Death* (Gateway Publications, 1989).

Levine, S., *Who Dies* (Gateway, 2000).

Neff, K., *Self-Compassion: Stop Beating Yourself Up and Leave Insecurity Behind* (HarperCollins, 2011).

Santorelli, S., *Heal Thy Self: Lessons on Mindfulness in Medicine* (Three Rivers Press, 2000).

Segal, Z., Williams, M., & Teasdale, J., *Mindfulness-based Cognitive Therapy for Depression: A New Approach for Preventing Relapse* (Guildford Press, 2002).

Smith, S., & Hayes, S., *Get Out of Your Mind and Into Your Life: The New Acceptance and Commitment Therapy* (New Harbinger Publications, 2005).

Williams, M., Segal, Z., Teasdale, J., & Kabat-Zinn J., *The Mindful Way Through Depression: Freeing Yourself from Chronic Unhappiness* (The Guildford Press, 2007).

MEDITATION AND MINDFULNESS

Analayo, Satipatthana, *The Direct Path to Realisation* (Windhorse Publications, 2003).

Bodhipaksa, *Wildmind: A Step-by-step Guide to Meditation* (Windhorse Publications, 2007).

Goldstein, J., *Insight Meditation: The Practice of Freedom* (Newleaf, 1994).

Goldstein, J., & Salzberg, S., *Insight Meditation: A step-by-step course on how to meditate (*Sounds True Inc. 2002).

Hart, W., *Vipassana Meditation: The Art of Living as Taught by S.N Goenka,* (HarperCollins, 1987).

Kabat-Zinn, J., *Wherever You Go, There You Are: Mindfulness Meditation in Everyday Life* (Piatkus 2004).

Kamalashila, *Meditation: Buddhist Way of Tranquillity and Insight* (Windhorse Publications, 2003).

Paramananda, *Change Your Mind* (Windhorse Publications, 1996).

Rosenberg, L., *Breath by Breath* (Thorsons, 1998).

Salzberg, S., *Lovingkindness: The Revolutionary Art of Happiness (*Shambhala Publications, 2004).

Sangharakshita, *Living with Awareness* (Windhorse Publications, 2003).

Tolle, E., *The Power of Now: A Guide to Spiritual Enlightenment* (Hodder, 2001).

Williams, M., & Kabat-Zinn, J., Mindfulness: Diverse Perspectives on its Meaning, Origins and Applications (Routledge, 2013).

ACCOUNTS OF MANAGING HEALTH DIFFICULTIES WITH AWARENESS OR MEDITATION

Bedard, J., *Lotus in the Fire: The Healing Power of Zen* (Shambhala Publications, 1999).

Bernhard, T., *How to be Sick* (Wisdom Publications, 2010).

Cohen, D., *Turning Suffering Inside Out: A Zen Approach to Living with Physical and Emotional Pain* (Shambhala Publications, 2003).

Rosenbaum, E., *Here for Now: Living Well with Cancer Through Mindfulness* (Satya House Publications, 2007).

Sadler, J., *Pain Relief without Drugs* (Healing Arts Press, 2007).

Sandford, M., *Waking: A Memoir of Trauma and Transcendence* (Rodale, 2006).

Shone, N., *Coping Successfully with Pain* (Sheldon Press, 1995).

PAIN

Bond, M., & Simpson, K., *Pain: Its Nature and Treatment* (Elsevier, 2006).

Cole, F., Macdonald, H., Carus, C., & Howden-Leach, H., *Overcoming Chronic Pain* (Constable & Robinson, 2005).

Nicholas, M., Molloy, A., Tonkin, L., & Beeston, L., *Manage Your Pain* (Souvenir Press, 2003).

Padfield, D., *Perceptions of Pain* (Dewi Lewis Publications, 2003).

Wall, P., *Pain: the Science of Suffering* (Columbia University Press, 2000).

Wall, P., & Melzack, R., *The Challenge of Pain* (Penguin Books, 1982).

APPENDIX

On the following pages you'll find the blank charts for you to photocopy and record your own information.

Daily activity diary

Date					
Time	**Activity**	**Time taken**	**Pain at end** (or whatever symptom you are scoring) **(1–10)**	**Tension at end (1–10)**	**0** (no change in pain or symptom) **+** (increase in pain or symptom) **–** (decrease in pain or symptom) **R** (rest)

Diary analysis sheet

+ **Extra pain** (or whatever symptom you have scored)	0 **No change in pain** (or whatever symptom you have scored)	– **Reduced pain** (or whatever symptom you have scored)

Rest period analysis sheet

Date	Length (mins/hours)	Total number	Total time

Baseline record for:

Baseline level:

Date	Level achieved	Notes

INDEX

(page numbers in italic type refer to illustrations)